COUNTDOWN TO COMMUNITY CARE

COUNTDOWN TO COMMUNITY CARE

Edited by
TRISH GROVES
Assistant editor, BMJ

With an introduction by
SIR ROY GRIFFITHS
*Deputy chairman, NHS policy board,
and former managing director of Sainsbury's*

Published by the BMJ Publishing Group
Tavistock Square, London WC1H 9JR

© BMJ Publishing Group 1993

All rights reserved. No part of this publication may be reproduced, stored in a retrieval system, or transmitted, in any form or by any means, electronic, mechanical, photocopying, recording and/or otherwise, without the prior written permission of the publishers.

First published 1993

British Library Cataloguing in Publication Data
A catalogue record for this book is available from the British Library

ISBN 0-7279-0790-5

The following picture sources are acknowledged:

Cover, pages 50, 53, 118, Sam Tanner; page 4, Sally and Richard Greenhill; page 13, Ulrike Preuss; pages 15, 107, 115, John Twinning; page 26, Age Concern Gwent; page 28, South Wales Argus; page 34, Frank Spooner/Gamma; pages 57, 60, City of Newcastle upon Tyne; page 63, North East Studios; page 71, Michael Mullen/Format; pages 91, 93, Mary Evans; page 108, Friern Hospital; page 101, Brenda Prince/Format.

Typeset by Bedford Typesetters Limited, Bedford
Printed and bound in Great Britain by
Latimer Trend & Company Ltd, Plymouth

Contents

	Page
Introduction	ix

ROY GRIFFITHS, *deputy chairman, NHS policy board, and former managing director of Sainsbury's*

Getting ready

Getting ready for change — 3
DAVID BROWNING, *associate director, health studies, Audit Commission, London SW1P 2PN*

What the changes mean — 12
TRISH GROVES, *assistant editor, BMJ*

Cross country view

Gwent: a head start in preparing for change — 21
ROGER ROBINSON, *associate editor, BMJ*

Bassetlaw: "The planning process has not been easy" — 32
TRISH GROVES, *assistant editor, BMJ*

Northern Ireland: building on integrated services — 43
ALISON TONKS, *assistant editor, BMJ*

Newcastle: "If it doesn't work here, it can't work anywhere" — 55
JANE SMITH, *deputy editor, BMJ*

Putting change into practice

Community care and the fundholder — 69
RHIDIAN MORRIS, *general practitioner, Ivybridge Health Centre, Ivybridge, Devon PL21 0AB*

Care management and mental health — 76
GRAHAM THORNICROFT, *senior lecturer, PRiSM (Psychiatric Research in Service Measurement), Institute of Psychiatry, London SE5 8AF;* PAUL WARD, *community and priority services contracts manager, South East London Commissioning Agency, London SE1 9RY;* STEVE JAMES, *community care coordinator, London Borough of Southwark, London SE1*

Community psychiatry in Scotland — 88
IAN PULLEN, *consultant psychiatrist, Royal Edinburgh Hospital, Edinburgh EH10 5HF*

	Page
Helping disabled people—the user's view	96
PETER SWAIN, *project leader, Living Options East Devon, Ashclyst Centre, Whipton, Exeter EX1 3RB*	
Mental health services—the user's view	105
PETER CAMPBELL, *freelance trainer of mental health workers, London NW2 2RG*	
Old people's homes—the relatives' view	113
MAVIS NICHOLSON, *journalist and broadcaster, Llanrhaeadr-Ym-Mochnant, Powys SY10 0AX;* DOROTHY WHITE, *chair, Relatives Association, London NW1 9PG*	
Index	121

ACKNOWLEDGMENTS

I would like to thank all the authors who contributed to *Countdown to Community Care*; Margaret Cooter, who did the technical editing; and Elaine Murphy, who helped us plan the series.

Introduction

This book is made up of a series of articles which have appeared in the *BMJ* in the past few months. As the author of the government report *Community Care—Agenda for Action* I read them with considerable interest even before being asked to write this foreword, but the request has sharpened my attention.

Timing may not be all but it is important. The book appears as the final stages of the legislation are being implemented and the act is fully enforced. The timing is right for other reasons. The 1980s was an unsympathetic decade for community care even though the amount spent by government had in fact increased sharply, largely owing to the social security payments for residential care. The 1980s' emphasis on competition and the individual was very necessary to bring the nation to the realities of survival, but the market became an end in itself with the words community and society being driven out of the political lexicon or at least out of ministerial documents. Times change, however. Recession alters not simply job prospects and the burden of mortgages but also one's beliefs. While emphasis on the individual and competition may be necessary to create wealth, an emphasis on the community and collaboration may be seen as even more necessary to use the wealth as created, or when the creation of wealth is faltering.

It was in December 1986 that the Audit Commission's report, *Making a Reality of Community Care*, dropped on to Norman Fowler's desk and he asked me to review the way in which public funds were used to support community care policy and to advise on the options for action that would improve the use of these funds as a contribution to more effective community care. My conclusions are well known and largely form the basis of the government legislation.

One or two recommendations were not obviously accepted. I suggested that government money for community care should be ring fenced. Two considerations led me to this recommendation. Firstly, a simple belief that if you are to hold people accountable then they need to be quite clear on three things: the work to be done; the timescale for achievement; and the money which is to be available. The second consideration was that, according to Treasury guidelines, the government is prepared to ring fence money for programmes of major national importance. I had assumed that community care fell within this category. The government finally did ring fence the money to be transferred from social security at least for a few years and also made specific ring fenced grants.

I also recommended that there should be a minister for community care. The simple objective was to give a higher profile to the subject. This objective was substantially achieved by the present secretary of state for health, whose professional background is in care in the community and who states that successful implementation of the legislation is her primary objective.

The major obstacle to acceptance of the recommendations was the lead role given to local government. In fact it already had the lead role, but the big change was to transfer the social security monies previously allocated to residential and nursing home care to local authorities, thus giving them a much larger budget and incidentally — and most importantly — allowing the rest of the act, with its emphasis on the individual and on carers and on people being looked after in the community, an opportunity to become a reality.

I had considered about eight alternatives but all were flawed and I was supported in my conclusions by a subsequent report by a heavyweight interdepartmental working committee. But again timing is important and the act comes into full force just as the government is encouraging better relationships between central government and the local authorities. If the bedraggled local government phoenix is accordingly to arise from the ashes of the 1980s and local government is really to be revitalised, it could be one of the most important and correct decisions of the present government.

It would be inappropriate for me in a brief foreword to comment specifically on each of the contributions. They illustrate the hopes and fears of those charged or affected by the changes. I can deal with one or two of the recurrent themes and offer some points of preliminary clarification.

First there is a major difference between the NHS and community care. Although there may be continuing arguments about the level of resources, the health service does aim to offer a reasonably comprehensive service, largely free at the point of delivery; in some cases the premises in which treatment is given may not be first class and there may be a wait for treatment, but nonetheless the objective is clear. With community care most of the social care is offered by relatives, and however high flown the philosophical discussion may be as to the divisional responsibilities among the family, the community, the authorities, and the government, the discussion always comes back to how the available resources are best used to support the individual and those, if any, caring for him or her. Priorities and targeting resources are always extremely difficult.

This comment leads me to the second point. I frequently see statements arising from detailed studies showing that, of the people in residential care, 75%-85% need to be there. My conclusion was not to disagree with these studies but simply to recognise that, of the resources available for community care, far too high a proportion was going to residential care—leaving too little for any attempt to look after people in their own homes.

The third point is the distinction between health and social care which is continually cited. This centres around the problems of discharge from hospitals and on who pays for the care subsequently provided. The distinction is accentuated by health care being free and by social care often being means tested. The distinction is not new and has largely been recognised and implemented previously, and it is on this basis that the government has left it to local discussion and clarification between the authorities involved.

Finally, there is a feeling by general practitioners that they have been involved only at a comparatively late stage of the initial preparations. The changes for general practitioners are not great, but what is needed is exactly what one of the general practitioner contributors emphasises—that when they do become involved in referring people to the social services it is done in an effective, disciplined way (as in the case of referrals to consultants) with written referral and follow up.

It is very important that in concentrating our gaze on the problems we do not lose sight of the opportunities and of the philosophy behind my original report. Many are worried that the work to establish the

INTRODUCTION

community care plans and the assessment procedures will throw up a lot of unmet need and the government will be found wanting. There is a lot of need in the community, but the real question is whose responsibility it is to meet that need. The thrust of my report was to recognise that need and to ask the local authorities to marshall all the resources of the community to meet that need as far as is consistent with the priorities as it sees them. All the resources of the community means not only of the statutory authorities but also the voluntary sector, employers, churches, and indeed individuals. Central government can help by opening up the debate as to how this can be achieved, including how people themselves can provide more of the care which they need in old age. Good pension schemes have been the hallmark of caring companies for the past fifty years. The thinking needs to move as to how companies can provide or adapt pension schemes for employees in the last stages of their life. The relationship of people in work to people of pensionable age is for the time being fairly constant. Even without recession and heavy unemployment the trend from the year 2000 will be to alter unfavourably that relationship. No government will commit itself to a heavy burden of social care, particularly at a time when the financial burden of health care will be increasingly onerous.

The various authorities will have had three years to think through the final implementation. This staged process of implementation has gone reasonably well, but the brave new world will reveal itself only gradually. What has been provided is a new framework and a new approach to delivery of a policy which has generally been government policy for the past thirty years. But the test over the rest of the decade is not simply of government legislation or of local authorities acceptability, but of the will of each of us as individuals and collectively to meet the needs of disadvantaged people in our society.

SIR ROY GRIFFITHS
April 1993

GETTING READY

Getting ready for change

DAVID BROWNING

In the past few years community care for elderly and disabled people has been moving steadily up the political agenda. At the 1992 conference of the Institute of Health Service Management, the secretary of state for health, Virginia Bottomley, announced it to be her top priority. The House of Commons health committee has made it one of three subjects for investigation in 1993 (together with dentistry and tobacco advertising). Dubbed the "Cinderella" service for so long, community care may be going to the ball at last. But before it can, those responsible must transform current arrangements into a fully integrated and well coordinated service—making the transformation for Cinders of a few mice, assorted lizards, and the odd pumpkin seem a relatively trivial task.

Community care services provide support for some of the most vulnerable members of society—mainly elderly people, but also people under 65 with physical disabilities, learning disabilities (formerly known as mental handicap), and long term mental illness.

The number of people needing such support is appreciable. In England and Wales by the end of this century there will be a million people aged over 85.[1] There are about half a million people below 65 with a significant physical handicap[2]; and there are about 125 000 adults with a significant learning disability[3] (although the numbers depend on how "significant" is defined). The number of people with long term mental health problems is notoriously difficult to estimate but is probably in six figures.

Social care is provided by local authorities and health care by community health services. But there is no neat dividing line between

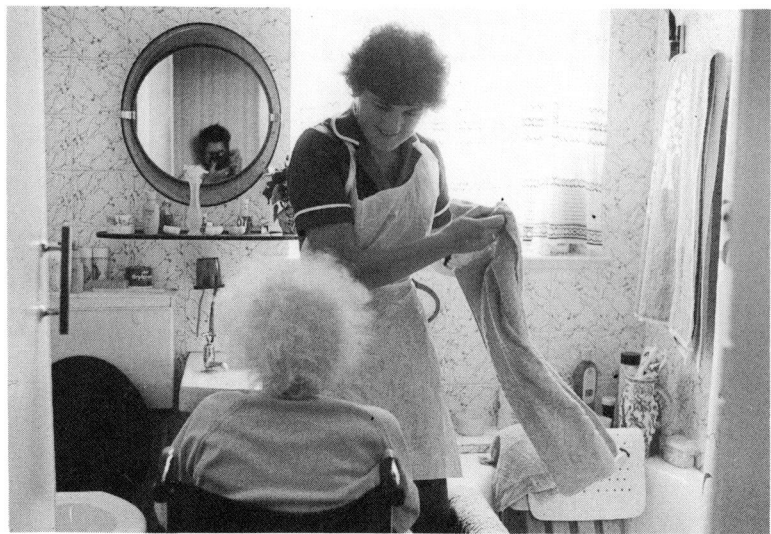

Who should run the bath—a health worker or a social worker?

social care and health care, and there has been much overlap and some buck passing at the margin. For example, there has been much debate about whether people who need help at home with bathing should receive "health baths" or "social baths." With general practice fundholders set to purchase community health from 1 April 1993, we may yet see the advent of the "practice bath" as a third option.

Community care has developed in a haphazard way, with little attention paid to its overall shape and direction. With responsibilities divided between authorities who have different priorities and traditions—and who may not even share the same geographical boundaries—it has been difficult to organise a coherent approach. The result too often has been muddle.[4]

The amount of home care, residential care, or district nursing available has always been as much an accident of history as any reflection of need. Levels of service have been relatively impervious to change because finance has always been provided en bloc from central government and budgets have been rolled over from year to year with no more than the occasional adjustment up or down at the margin. Potential users of community care have been assessed against set criteria for each service, and those trying to meet people's needs have always had to fit them into whatever range of services happened to be available. The overall effect has been to produce a pattern of care which is often disjointed and dominated by the requirements of services rather than by the needs of users.

Pressures on the NHS have been building as the numbers of long stay beds and the lengths of stay of people in acute beds have been reducing, further increasing the numbers requiring community care. The resulting shortfall has been filled by growing numbers of private nursing and residential homes[5] funded by social security benefits (figure)—prompting some to say that a considerable part of the NHS has now been privatised.[6] The suitability (not to mention the cost) of this form of care, allegedly sometimes provided without the satisfactory consideration of alternatives, has been questioned by many—not least by the Treasury, which has been picking up the bill.

Putting people first

All of this is now set to change. The 1990 NHS and Community

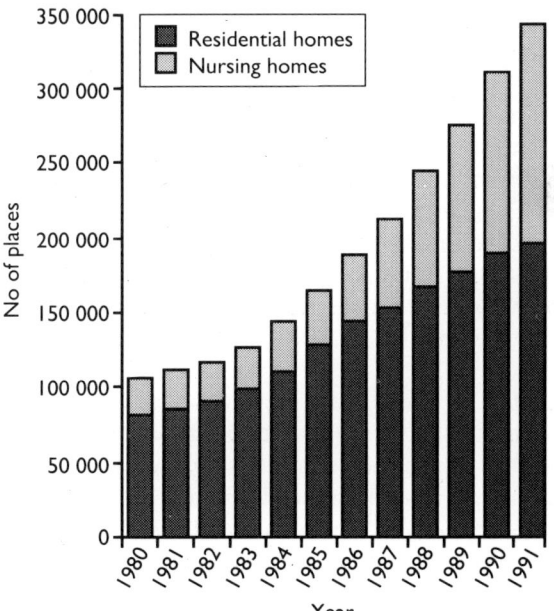

Residential and nursing homes in the independent sector, United Kingdom. From *Laing's Review of Private Health Care 1991/2*

Care Act, which came into force in full on 1 April 1993, introduces a fundamentally different approach. Its main aim for community care is to put the needs of service users and carers first. It gives lead responsibility to local authorities, transferring to them over a period of years much of the finance that is now going in social security payments to users of private homes.[7]

This change in emphasis from services to users and their carers will require many other changes.[8] Authorities will need to start formulating eligibility criteria to decide who is to receive help and who is not; and they must decide how much help people should receive. This will force them to go back to basics: looking at patterns of need, calculating the resource implications of those needs, and adjusting eligibility criteria so that budgets are not exceeded. These basic rationing decisions will cause great difficulties for many local authorities, requiring some hard decisions on priorities.

Doctors and others within the NHS have a major interest in this process. Community care is inextricably linked with both primary and secondary care. If community care does not operate in consort with both, the NHS could quickly become overloaded with people requiring support but with nowhere to go. At present many hospital beds are occupied by people no longer needing medical care who are simply waiting for suitable arrangements for discharge. General practitioners' surgeries are packed with people whose real needs are for support rather than medical attention.

If local authorities' priorities do not mesh with those of the NHS, then these sorts of difficulties will grow. It is more important than ever that the NHS and local authorities should sit down and plan together. A drive by a health authority or trust to increase the number of hip replacements, for example, will fail if suitable arrangements for support afterwards are not planned at the same time.

Plans and priorities

All local authorities are required to produce a community care plan setting out their priorities and all must consult with other agencies, including district health authorities and family health services authorities—who should in turn consult with local authorities on their plans. There should, therefore, be a framework in place for authorities to coordinate priorities.

But if this framework is to work a number of long standing problems will need to be addressed. How will local authorities with locally elected members, committees, and committee cycles coordinate their decision making with health authorities that have such new management cultures? What will happen when the priorities of one authority do not match those of another? In particular, what will happen if one authority's priorities require another to spend more money?

Whatever strategic solutions are worked out, clear definitions will be needed, setting out which people qualify for help, so that general practitioners, other health workers, and social workers all know how to work the new arrangements without wasting each other's time. In particular, assessments by local authority staff will have to be undertaken in conjunction with health staff if they are to provide a balanced picture. Many of the more dependent users of services will require both health and social care, and many tend to approach their general practitioners first when they require either form of care. In November 1992 the Department of Health circulated guidelines to general practitioners on the subject of assessment for social care.[9] The success of the community care policy will depend ultimately on practitioners from all authorities making it work at the sharp end.

Care management

To strengthen coordination between practioners the reforms promote the concept of the "care manager," who is to be the social care equivalent of the general practitioner fundholder. Funds are to be devolved to care managers, who will coordinate the assessment process, provide advice on possible services, and arrange (and, where appropriate, pay for) services as necessary.

As yet, care management is not widely available and it will probably follow some time after the initial reforms. Many authorities have pilot projects underway, but the usual problems of converting pilot projects to mainstream practice apply. Some authorities seem to oppose the concept altogether, while others are trying out different models. In some situations care managers are being based in general practitioners' surgeries, forging closer links with general practitioners and primary health care teams. Perhaps this will bring the concept of the "one stop health care shop" closer to reality. This concept envisages all social and health care coordinated under one roof—with professionals who know each other sorting out the professional boundary disputes together, within the policy framework set by health and local authorities.

Making it work

Just as there will be difficulties coordinating strategic priorities, a number of knotty local problems will need to be unravelled if these arrangements are to work. It is not clear who will coordinate professionals locally or who will deal with disputes. Perhaps community care teams will be loose federations, as many primary health care teams are now. General practitioners may be suitable team leaders but will then have little time for patients. And how will general practitioner fundholders fit in?

The success of care management will depend not only on such local organisational arrangements but also on the resources available, the quality of people appointed to the job, the support they are given, and the policy framework within which they operate. At first, resources will probably be limited, with most still locked up in existing services. But over time, more money should become available, albeit at different rates in different areas of the country.

The evidence suggests that, where real choice is available, the

---

Case report: Mr John H; age 47; multiple sclerosis

Mr H had advanced MS, was confined to bed with a catheter, and could hardly speak. He choked easily and was prone to sudden infections, so his wife felt that whoever was to give her a break by providing care for him must have nursing experience.

For a few months before the Independent Living Fund award, a care assistant recommended by Crossroads had been employed for three hours a week plus one night to give Mrs H one good night's sleep. The ILF money had enabled her to extend that to seven daytime hours and two nights a week.

"Seven hours to yourself in the week. Seven hours out of 168 gets your head showered."

Mrs H saw the second night as a means of avoiding exhaustion. She had stopped respite care in hospital for her husband because there had been feeding problems and he had developed pressure sores. She was confident that with a bit of help to keep her going, she could provide better care for him at home. Care is "not a big handful if I have help."

Between April and September, social services had also increased the amount of domestic help provided for the H's from five to seven hours, and overall Mrs H felt that care arrangements were working very well for the two of them. Her only regret was that she did not apply to the ILF some time ago when she first heard of it. Getting the award earlier could have prevented a period of extreme exhaustion and distress.[10]

services selected by care managers are very different from the traditional ones. The Independent Living Fund, set up to plug a loophole in the social security system, provides service users and their carers with cash for care. The resulting patterns of care often involve neighbours and friends paid to come in at odd hours, rather than day centres and residential care (see box).[10] Equally, where care managers have been given real discretion, exciting new initiatives are reported to be emerging. The benefits of the new approach seem real, if difficult to realise.

To give greater choice, care managers should be able to buy services from other agencies, so that local authorities do not continue to provide everything for themselves. Many services in the community are best provided by the community itself rather than by the local council, no matter how well motivated the staff.

Care managers are being recruited from a variety of backgrounds, including teaching and nursing, and not just from social work. The skills required include good organisational abilities, not only the more traditional caring skills. Certainly, care management will have to be supported by suitable financial controls and by information systems which have yet to be developed, and those taking on the job must be trained to use them effectively.

Where hospital doctors fit in

In case hospital doctors are feeling very pleased that they are not involved in all of this, the changes keep the biggest potential sting for them. One of the major changes introduced by the 1990 act is the transfer of funds previously available through the social security system for residential and nursing home places in the private sector to local authorities. Placement of people with limited financial means will, from 1 April 1993, be at the discretion of social services; and the amount of money available (£399m in 1993-4 in England) will be cash limited.

Surveys suggest that 250-500 people a year are being placed directly into private homes from an average district general hospital. Though this is not a large number, any failure to make suitable arrangements for discharge with local authorities could increase lengths of stay appreciably, with a knock on effect on the availability of beds and the number of patients treated (with financial implications for trusts) and ultimately on waiting lists, which are seen to be a key indicator of performance.

It will therefore be even more essential to negotiate appropriate discharge arrangements for patients. This will be a two way process requiring changes in practice in hospitals as well as in social services. In some situations, patients may have been placed in nursing homes as quickly as possible to clear beds without a full assessment of all the options. In future it may be necessary to allow a little more time for proper assessment, with corresponding improvements in the quality of care given. If this creates difficulties because of pressure on beds then interim convalescent arrangements may be necessary while longer term decisions are made. (Hotels are used in the United States, but short term places in nursing homes would serve as well, and possibly better.)

There is much useful guidance on hospital discharge arrangements,[11] and it will be important to follow good practice and, if necessary, fund improvements. Any interim arrangements could be funded by both health and social services—concentrating both sets of minds on quick but appropriate solutions. Quite apart from the logistics, the sensitive handling of the difficult transition out of hospital is a crucial part of successful patient care. Certainly, hospital discharge arrangements will provide an early indicator of how well the new community care arrangements are working.

Timetable for change

Local authorities are now pressing on with preparations for the changes although, inevitably, there are some who are making more progress than others, prompting the formation of a national "support force" to provide advice and promote good practice.

The implementation of the changes in full at both strategic and operational levels will take many years, and the targets for 1 April 1993 are relatively modest. Health and local authorities must be able to coordinate assessments, especially for discharge from hospital. They must have in place suitable financial arrangements for managing the funds transferred from social security. Finally, they must have negotiated suitable arrangements with private residential and nursing homes, with a requirement to spend at least 85% of the extra money transferred on services not supplied by local authorities. The more profound changes, such as care management, can be planned at a more leisurely pace.

The theory is now mostly in place, with copious guidance from the centre; authorities and practitioners must now make it work. The early signs are that where it works it is worth all the effort, with better patterns of care emerging and a higher quality of life for some of the most disadvantaged members of society. But community care is not an easy or particularly cheap option.

With increasing emphasis on efficiency and best use of scare resources, requiring ever shorter lengths of stay and more rationing, the smooth functioning of the rest of the NHS depends increasingly on suitable provision for long term care. Community care is now the main method of providing such care. It is up to everyone to make it work through better assessments, better hospital discharge arrangements, and better cooperation and organisation all round. Failure to do so could mean that the Cinderella services arrive at the ball still in tatters, with profound implications for the NHS and local government alike.

1 National population projections: mid 1989-based. *OPCS Monitor* 1991;**1**. (PP2 91/1.)
2 Beardshaw V. *Last on the list: community services for people with physical disabilities.* London: King's Fund Institute, 1988.
3 Audit Commission. *Developing community care for adults with a mental handicap.* London: HMSO, 1989. (Occasional paper No 9.)
4 Audit Commission. *Making a reality of community care.* London: HMSO, 1986.
5 *Laing's Review of Private Health Care 1991/2.* London: Laing and Buisson Publications, 1992.
6 Harrison A. Commentary. In: *Health Care UK 1991.* London: King's Fund Institute, 1992.
7 Secretaries of State for Health, Social Security, Wales, and Scotland. *Caring for people: community care in the next decade and beyond.* London: HMSO, 1989. (Cm 849.)
8 Audit Commission. *Managing the cascade of change.* London: HMSO, 1992.
9 Department of Health. *General practitioners and caring for people.* London: DoH, 1992.
10 Kestenbaum A. *Cash for care: a report on the experience of Independent Living Fund clients.* London: Independent Living Fund, 1992.
11 Department of Health. *Discharge of patients from hospital.* London: DoH, 1989. (HC (89)5.)

What the changes mean

TRISH GROVES

For many years now the British government has tried to replace institutional care with community care, particularly for people with chronic mental illness and learning disability (mental handicap). According to some researchers, this quest for "normalisation" has had too high a price, leaving many former patients untreated on our city streets. At the same time, many old people who might have coped in their own homes with adequate support have been sent to residential homes, at great expense to the tax payer. Whether or not the government believes that community care has failed thus far, it has listened to the criticisms and decided to overhaul its policy.

New ways of delivering and funding care are being introduced. But, as David Browning of the Audit Commission has already pointed out, this will probably bring evolution rather than revolution. Unlike the sweeping reforms that hospital staff and general practitioners have had to cope with in the past few years, the changes to community care are being introduced more gently.

Time to think again

In theory, gradual change should have allowed doctors time to think about and understand the community care reforms. Yet many doctors still find the plans confusing and nebulous, not least because many of the changes seem relevant only to social workers and health service managers. The jargon terms that pop up in community care literature—"user," "mixed economy," "needs-led," and "ring fencing"—are off putting. And even the term "community care" seems ambiguous at times. Does it include community health services—those paramedical and nursing services such as occupational therapy, chiropody, and district nursing? And aren't these part of primary care?

When policy makers and planners talk about community care they are not usually referring to community health or primary care services. Instead, they mean practical and social services for people who need help with daily life but are not so disabled that they have to live in large institutions and hospitals. Most people who need such help can be fitted conveniently into discrete groups: they are frail and old, or have chronic psychiatric problems, or have mental or physical handicaps.

Some critics argue, however, that lumping disadvantaged people into labelled groups and assuming that they all have roughly the same needs is patronising and stigmatising. Trying to make people match existing services can also lead to failure to provide the right kind or amount of care. When too little care is given, people's needs are not met. When too much is given (for instance, when elderly patients are sent unnecessarily to residential homes), people's rights are ignored and scarce time and money are wasted.

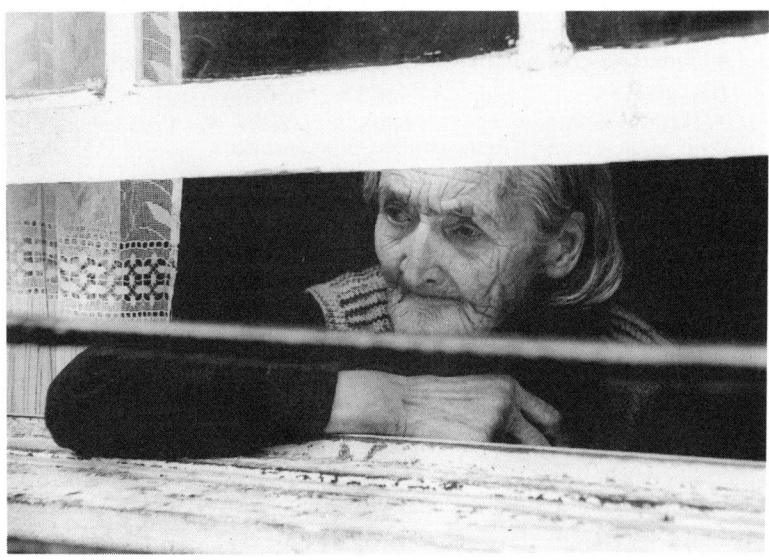

Waiting for the revolution

Radical change required

One of the first critiques of this "service led" community care system came from the Audit Commission. The commission is an independent body that was established nearly 10 years ago to monitor the economics, efficiency, and effectiveness of public services. In 1986 it reviewed community care and found much of it to be seriously uneconomic, inefficient, and ineffective.[1] Following this the government decided to set up its own review and asked Sir Roy Griffiths, deputy chairman of both the NHS policy board and the Sainsbury's supermarket chain, to execute it.

The Griffiths report, published in 1988, suggested radical changes to community care.[2] Local authorities should act as brokers of care by assessing people's needs and buying them packages of services, said

---

Countdown to community care

April 1991
- Inspection and complaints procedures set up
- Grants for severe mental illness and drug and alcohol problems introduced

April 1992
- Community care plans published by local authorities after consulting health authorities, family health services authorities, and other agencies
- Care programmes introduced for severely mentally ill people

December 1992
- Health authorities (health boards in Scotland) draw up plans on good practice in discharging patients from hospital

April 1993
- Local authorities take lead responsibility and receive funding for strategic purchasing and care management
- Care management starts
- User and carers get more say in planning, assessment, and choice of services, and can complain more easily
- General practitioners get regular information about local care services, make prompt and effective referrals for care, and provide basic clinical information to care managers (with patients' permission)
- Community care plans and services are monitored by local inspection units and the Social Services Inspectorate.

These details apply in England, Wales, and Scotland. In Northern Ireland health and social services already work together in boards which will fund and organise care management after April 1993.

WHAT THE CHANGES MEAN

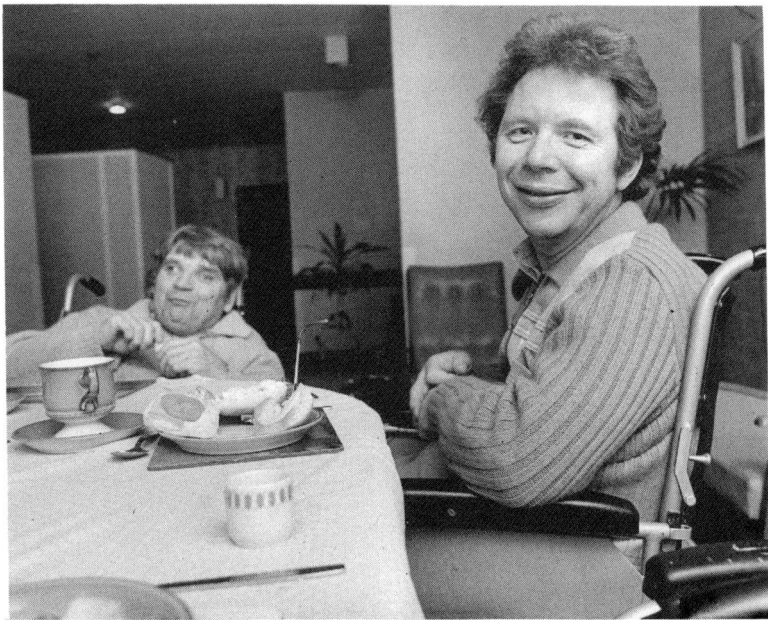

Users of community care will get more say if all goes to plan

Sir Roy. Clearly earmarked or "ring fenced" funds to do this should be raised by stopping social security payments for residential care and giving the money to local authorities. Care packages should include services run by the independent (private and voluntary) sector as well as statutory social services, drawing together a haphazard collection of services to make an accessible and usable "mixed economy" of care. Finally, a minister for community care should be appointed to coordinate the various government departments—including health, social security, education, and environment—that play a part in delivering care.

The government agreed to implement most of Sir Roy's recommendations,[3,4] and, after several delays and setbacks,[5] set April 1993 as the full starting date. There will be no minister for community care, however, and funds will be earmarked only for a three year transitional period.[6]

What will happen when

Some of the changes have happened already. Mechanisms for

planning, inspecting, and complaining about the new system have been introduced over the past two years.

In addition, to quell mounting fears about psychiatric community care, three measures directly affecting people with mental health problems have begun. The first two measures are special grants for which local authorities and voluntary organisations must bid. One is designed to help the voluntary sector (organisations such as Turning Point and Alcohol Concern) to develop services for people with drug and alcohol problems. The other is meant to fund new services for people with severe mental illness. The third measure is the introduction of care programmes. Since April 1991 health authorities have had to ensure that patients with severe mental illness are offered comprehensive and well documented programmes of care on discharge from hospital. Patients must be allocated named key workers and care must be supervised and reviewed continuously by consultant psychiatrists.

Managing care

Sarah Jarvis is a 72 year old widow who has spent the past three months in hospital after having a stroke. Despite some residual weakness on the left side she can just about walk with a Zimmer frame. She is eager to get home and her consultant agrees that hospital care is no longer necessary.

Mrs Jarvis's medical team has referred her to the local social services department and she has been allocated a care manager, Judy Peters. She hasn't met Judy, but she knows how to contact her if any problems arise. Several people have come to the hospital to find out what help she will need after discharge. Her key worker, Jim Grant, has taken her back home with an occupational therapist and a home help organiser to assess what aids she might need.

Mrs Jarvis's general practitioner, Dr Harley, already knows that discharge is imminent and has a fair idea of the help being organised, because the ward sister has phoned the practice nurse to explain the plan. In addition Dr Harley has spoken to Judy Peters about Mrs Jarvis's general health (with permission, of course) and has asked a district nurse to provide help with bathing.

As soon as some ramps and safety rails have been fitted around the house, Mrs Jarvis will be discharged. Because she won't be able to get out and about on her own, she has been offered a place at the local Age Concern day centre twice a week, plus a lift there from a volunteer driver.

Care management

April 1993 sees the arrival of the most radical changes and of a new breed of professional. Care managers (who will probably have trained and worked as social workers, home care organisers, community nurses, or other practitioners) are roughly the social services equivalent of fundholding general practitioners. Unlike general practitioners, however, care managers will not actually deliver care themselves. Rather, they will organise multidisciplinary assessments for people needing help and will then try to arrange exactly what is needed. A case vignette is probably the easiest way to illustrate care management (see box).

The idea, as the Department of Health puts it, is "to respond flexibly and sensitively to the needs of users and their carers; allow a range of options; intervene no more than is necessary to foster independence; prevent deterioration; and concentrate on those with the greatest needs." The idea is good. But many commentators, including the BMA[7] and the Audit Commission,[8] still worry that putting it into practice will prove too difficult.

1 Audit Commission. *Making a reality of community care*. London: HMSO, 1986.
2 Griffiths R. *Community care: agenda for action*. London: HMSO, 1988.
3 Secretaries of State for Health, Social Security, Wales, and Scotland. *Caring for people: community care in the next decade and beyond*. London: HMSO, 1989.
4 Secretary of State for Northern Ireland. *People first, community care in Northern Ireland in the 1990s*. London: HMSO, 1990. (Cm 849.)
5 Murphy E. *After the asylums: community care for people with mental illness*. London: Faber and Faber, 1991.
6 Department of Health. *Caring for people newsletter* 1992;**11**.
7 British Medical Association. *Priorities for community care*. London: BMA, 1992.
8 Audit Commission. *The community care revolution: personal social services and community care*. London: HMSO, 1992.

CROSS COUNTRY VIEW

Gwent: a head start in preparing for change

ROGER ROBINSON

Gwent is a county of geographical and social variety. It includes Blaenau Gwent in the north, an old mining valley area whose pits had all shut down before the recent wholesale proposals for closure; Newport in the south, with some inner city problems; and Monmouth in the east, a large, sparsely populated area of rich farming country.

Gwent has had a head start in preparing for change. In many ways it has been progressive in planning and providing community care. For the past nine years the county has followed the All-Wales Strategy for Mental Handicap (this term is still used instead of learning disability in the title of the scheme),[1] setting up a community based system of care with assessment and planning centred on individual needs. The All-Wales Strategy for Mental Illness has been implemented more recently.[2] Planning is easier than in many counties because the boundaries of local authorities and health authorities coincide. There is a strong and active voluntary sector. Finally, the Welsh Office is responsible for both health and social services.

I spent three days in Gwent talking to some of the people who are planning the new way of community care or who will be affected by it. What follows is a series of impressions which do not necessarily apply throughout the county, or represent generally the attitudes of each interested group, but do indicate what some of those involved in the new plans are thinking and doing.

The planners

Social services

"This is the biggest change to have hit social services departments

GWENT: A HEAD START IN PREPARING FOR CHANGE

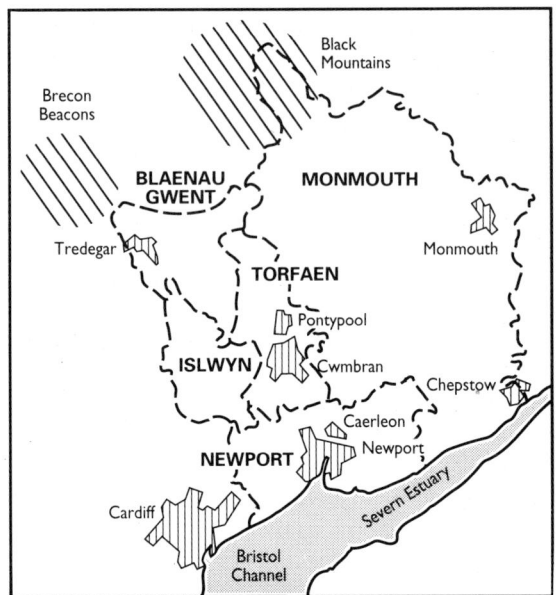

Gwent has five boroughs and great social and geographical variety

since they started," says Paul Meredith, principal planning officer of Gwent County Council's social service department. He is in no doubt of the scale or importance of the changes in community care, nor of their benefit to the users in the long run. He distinguishes, however, between those statutory changes which must happen by 1 April and those, such as the introduction of care management, which will come in more gradually.

Of the statutory changes, the one causing most general anxiety is the transfer to social services of the social security funds that are now spent on residential and nursing home care. Paul Meredith thinks that this change will force difficult decisions in Gwent, where there has been a huge increase recently in private nursing home placements of elderly people funded by social security. Nearly four fifths of private residential provision in Gwent is in nursing homes, compared with two fifths in the rest of the country. Furthermore, a survey of people in residential care in Gwent showed that those in private nursing homes had very similar levels of dependency to those in local authority (non-nursing) residential homes. Although Mr Meredith is cautious about deriving any conclusions from these statistics, he wonders whether the new assessment and funding procedures may lead to less use of nursing homes in future. He is clear that the transferred funds will not cover the use of private nursing homes if the homes continue to proliferate at the present rate.

Planning for implementing the community care legislation in Wales differs from that in England, in that the user groups targeted do not include those with mental illness or learning disability. Structures of care and some ring fenced funds already exist for them. Chronically and terminally ill people, however, and those who misuse drugs or alcohol, are added to the user groups. Informal carers are not specified as a distinct user group, but their importance is emphasised.

Each of the five boroughs of Gwent has an "area forum" with representatives of health and social services, users, carers, and the voluntary sector. These forums aim to review local community care, advise on developments, and monitor how the service operates. There are also three county based working groups responsible for assessment and care management, training, and accommodation.[3]

The final pattern for the new community care arrangements throughout Gwent will depend partly on the outcome of two pilot projects in assessment and care management. These projects are running in two very different social settings—Tredegar, a former mining community with high levels of unemployment, and Monmouth, a relatively affluent country town.

Mrs Joyce Steven, assistant county treasurer, is chair of the Joint Care Planning Board—the master interagency committee responsible for community care plans. She says that decisions on payments for residential care will be taken initially by planners in County Hall and will be devolved to local teams when there is some experience of how the new system works. The social services department is against making block contracts for care with proprietors of private nursing homes, though that is what the proprietors want. Mrs Steven does not foresee any sudden change in care arrangements on 1 April, and says, "In the initial period, the current pattern will have to be largely preserved."

Mrs Steven thinks that financial flexibility will be very limited at first, although she hopes some money will be freed for new initiatives and developments. Looking further ahead, she wonders if a lot of unmet need will come to light as the new assessment procedures begin to work. From the experience of the strategy for people with learning disabilities, she thinks that the families who will benefit least are those who seem to be coping.

Health services

A joint directorate and joint planning executive have been formed by Gwent Health Authority and Gwent Family Health Services Authority. Perry Williams, whom I met at headquarters at Pontypool with his assistant Julie Mullins, is the joint planning director. They explained that Wales had a "strategic intent and direction" policy for health, in advance of *The Health of the Nation*,[4] and that Gwent had developed its own health strategy.[5] A shift towards prevention and from secondary to primary care is planned, moving some outpatient and follow up care nearer to the patient's home—for example, to general practice. To support this change, 15% of funds are to move from the hospital service to primary care over three years. These developments have an obvious bearing on community care plans.

Mr Williams and Ms Mullins believe that health screening of people over 75, required by the general practitioner contract, could be a useful part of the new assessment structure and they are prepared to direct money to encourage training for this purpose. They point out that for many clients the general practitioner is, and will remain, the point of entry to whatever new community care arrangements are made. They emphasise that health planners have good relations with those in the local authority, and have no major anxieties about how community care will develop.

Service providers and users

Testing the new methods

The pilot project in Tredegar, mentioned above, has been running for just over a year. Caroline Lewis, the senior social worker organising the project, told me that it has three main aims—to establish an area forum, to set up interagency training of all those who will work the new system, and to develop the new assessment procedures.

One initial problem was finding users and carers to serve on the area forum; Tredegar has many fewer voluntary workers than other parts of Gwent. On assessment Ms Lewis said, "We had to go back a few paces and think out the philosophies first"—in other words, the project team had to think through the idea of needs led assessment rather than begin by choosing particular methods of assessment. Now that the system is up and running the team has started using, and is enthusiastic about, an interactive computer program, TEC-SYS, developed by Bath University to assist assessment and care manage ent. It stores information on clients' changing needs and on available resources and helps to match them.

Ms Lewis has a budget of £20 000 for innovative ways of enabling people to stay in the community rather than go into residential care. Previously it was very unusual for a senior social worker to have a flexible budget of this kind, and she has found it immensely useful for meeting individual needs in individual ways. For example, an elderly woman was on the brink of accepting residential care even though it was not what she really wanted. Providing money for transport for day care twice a week gave her the extra support she needed to remain at home.

Ms Lewis believes that there are substantial unmet needs in the community and thinks that the process of referral—how those in need actually reach the point of having their needs assessed—should be another important aspect of future plans.

Psychiatry and psychogeriatrics

In southern Gwent a huge shift towards community care for the mentally ill happened long before either the new legislation or the All-Wales Strategy for Mental Illness. St Cadoc's at Caerleon is a large mental illness hospital, whose original 700 beds have been reduced over the past 20 years to 68 acute and 10 long stay beds, with further reductions planned.

Dr Stephen Hunter, consultant in psychological medicine, and Dr Nick Warner, psychogeriatrician, give credit for this change mainly to their predecessors. They emphasise the value in community care of community psychiatric nurses and the voluntary sector, such as the local branches of the national association for mental health, MIND. Dr Hunter points out that, in the early years, the money saved by closing beds disappeared into other parts of the hospital service. In the past five years, however, all the savings have gone into community provision—for example, of the vitally important community psychiatric nurses.

Neither consultant expects major difficulties in delivering care under the new system. Dr Hunter has some anxiety that it may be less easy to arrange care for schizophrenic patients leaving acute psychiatric wards. Around one in 20 of these patients will have continuing problems needing community care, and he hopes that a system which has worked well for a long time will not be interfered with. He is worried "on a scale of 3 or 4 out of 10."

Dr Warner is a professed optimist. He does not want assessments done in the psychogeriatric unit to be duplicated in the community, but he has good working relationships with colleagues in social services and says that no one will want to interfere with a system which is working well. "I have never had any problem getting what I want for a patient," he asserts, although both he and Dr Hunter wonder whether the new system will be able to respond to the increasing number of elderly people with dementia and their carers.

Peter Clark is a community psychiatric nurse working in a multidisciplinary team in the Cwmbran area. The proposed changes in April have not yet made any special impact on Mr Clark's work and he expects no great changes in the way his team functions. But he is worried about existing resources and says that young mentally ill people often have needs, such as more help at home or more day care facilities, which the available funds do not meet. As an example of the frustration that the team feels over this, members sometimes spend a weekend cleaning or decorating a patient's flat.

Geriatrics

St Woolos Hospital, near the centre of Newport, is a recently extended former workhouse building with 170 beds for care of elderly people, a day unit, and assessment facilities. I met Dr Ann Freeman,

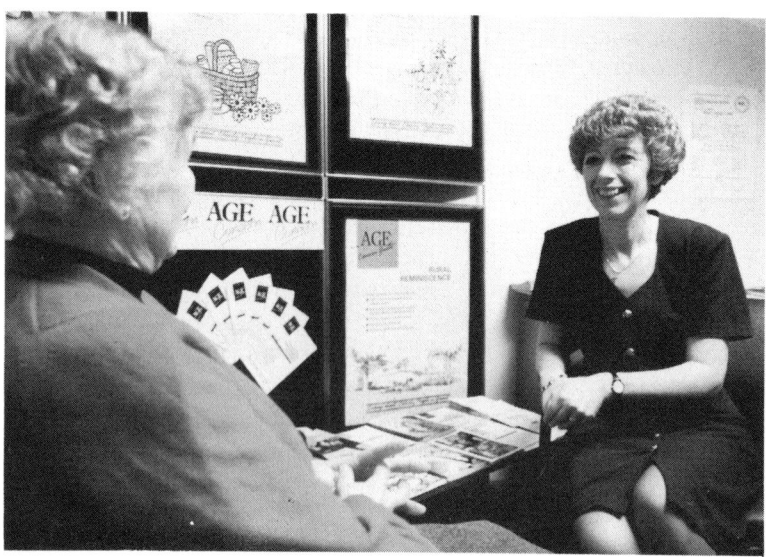

The voluntary sector is a key player in the plans for community care

the consultant geriatrician, Professor John Pathy and Dr Jan Beynon from the associated research unit, and Susan Burnett, the business manager. They all have definite anxieties about the effect of the community care changes, particularly in relation to discharge from hospital.

The new procedures for assessment might increase pressure on hospital beds, causing delays in discharge and leading to increased lengths of stay. The St Woolos team members feel strongly that the detailed assessments which they do should be accepted for this purpose and would also be very happy for the day hospital facilities to be used for assessments from the community. Although local social workers have had good relationships with the team, they often had to repeat the assessments. Professor Pathy believes that there should be central guidance on the nature of the new assessments, pointing out that validated measures and scales are available.

The voluntary sector

At Age Concern Gwent in Newport I spoke to Jane Reeks, the organiser. Her office now has a budget of £200 000 per year, some of which comes from the Welsh Office and the health authority and some from social services. Age Concern uses some paid coordinators and support workers, as well as large numbers of volunteers.

Age Concern is running two important schemes in community care in Gwent. One, worked out in cooperation with the geriatric teams, supports patients discharged home from hospital. Paid support workers give intensive help immediately after discharge, then voluntary workers are used, gradually tailing off to prevent the users becoming too dependent. The second scheme is a "home-from-home" service to give relief to carers by offering the elderly person respite care with a host family for a short period. Age Concern hopes to be able to arrange 200 placements of this kind each year.

Ms Reeks has some anxieties about the community care changes. The implications of making contracts with care managers to provide help for elderly people have not yet been worked out. She is worried that the funds available to social services departments will not be adequate to meet all needs, that there may be more emphasis on dealing with crises than on prevention, and that the new assessment procedures may introduce rigidity and delay.

General practice

The general practitioners I visited feel overwhelmed by the

problems of coping with the changes of the past three years—both of the new contract and of becoming fundholders. The community care changes seem to them remote and rather theoretical. Dr Peter Jones and Dr Julian Costello belong to a fundholding practice with six partners, operating from purpose built premises in an underprivileged area of Newport.

Both doctors have had to put enormous effort into reaching targets—for example, for immunisation. They feel no enthusiasm for the screening of their 500 patients over 75, an activity whose value they doubt. They do not feel they have an easy working relationship with social services, who seem available only for crisis intervention. In geriatrics and psychogeriatrics, however, these general practitioners feel that the service provided through the consultants is so good that contingent social problems will be looked after.

There must be other practices with similar problems and attitudes in Gwent. Dr Freeman, the consultant geriatrician, had a disappoint-

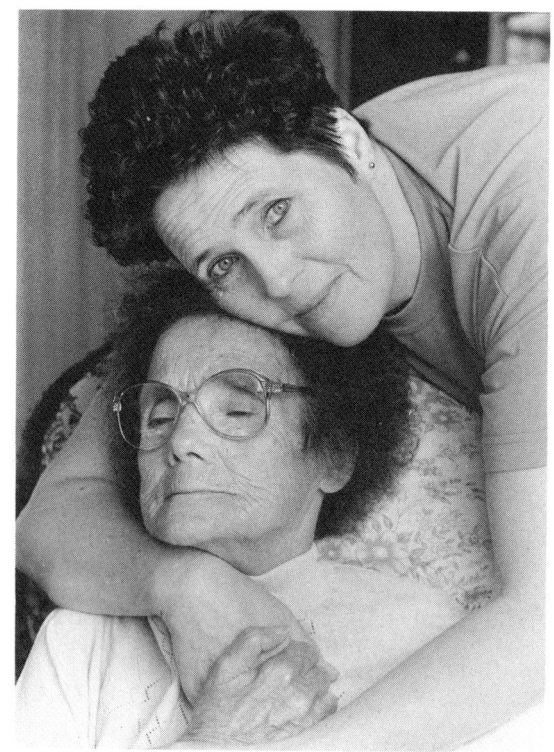

Would Mrs May have got more help to look after her mother under the new community care system?

ing response when she invited general practitioners to a symposium on screening people over 75. She also confirmed that some, but not all, general practitioners are happy to leave the arrangements for social care of elderly people to the geriatricians.

Informal carers

Mrs Ann May cared for her mother with Alzheimer's disease for four years until she died at home 18 months ago. Believing her mother had left her a legacy of knowledge and skill, Mrs May found herself increasingly involved in counselling other carers, providing a telephone support line, and working for several voluntary groups. Recently she has talked at training days for social workers and other professionals and has represented carers on several committees, including the Joint Care Planning Board. She came to these last activities with no previous experience and at first felt lost in the committee jargon and procedures.

Mrs May speaks of the enormous burden and financial cost for carers. "We are disabled ourselves by it," she says. She is hopeful about the new community care plans, but expects no great and immediate changes, which she thinks will take a decade to happen. Mrs May lives with her husband in a small house on the outskirts of Newport and works from a tiny office attached to the house. The office used to be the kennel where she bred Yorkshire terriers until her involvement in caring and carers forced her to give that up. Mrs May has provided her own computer and learned to use it herself, and her work is unpaid except for lecture fees and some travelling expenses.

Common themes

Several of the people I saw expressed concern that there may be a lot of unseen and therefore unmet need for community care, and that if this does get recognised by the new procedures—as it should—the resources will be even more stretched than expected. Two projects, however, argue against a huge pool of unrecognised need.

Dr Warner and his colleagues in psychogeriatrics advertised widely to offer a service to people who had memory problems or knew someone in the family who had them. He had some trepidation about the likely size of the response and the team's ability to cope; in fact the response was very small.

Professor Pathy's team did a pilot project on screening people over 65 for health and other problems.[6] They found about half needing a home visit or some form of referral, but did not uncover a great deal of unmet social need of a kind likely to place a major burden on the community services. On the other hand, the pilot project in Tredegar (which may represent a special social situation) has suggested significant unmet needs.

A central principle of the new style community care is that it should be needs led rather than service led. This principle was strongly held by social service planners and by the Tredegar pilot project, but rarely mentioned by others. There may have been a very good reason for this—most of the people to whom I spoke were so clearly orientated to patients' or clients' needs in their activities and plans that the principle had no novelty.

In one area—the meals-on-wheels service—a move to a needs led service might be expected to help. Mr Clark told me that some of the patients looked after by the community psychiatric team could be helped by this service, but that it is available only to people over 65. Dr Beynon told me that the rules for obtaining the service are so stringent that the team involved in the elderly screening project knew it was often not worth requesting it. This seemed a clear example of a service led activity which should be needs led, but no one seemed to expect that the new structure would solve this problem.

Conclusion

The overall impression in Gwent was of a community advanced in its thinking and practice about community care, with several schemes in operation before the new legislation starts. Nevertheless, the detailed plans for the new structure still need a good deal of filling in.

Most people I met were less bullish than the Audit Commission about the benefits of the new structure for community care, and few, except to some extent among the planners, regarded the changes as a revolution or major upheaval. Nearly everyone spoke well of the cooperation between health, social services, and the voluntary sector. There is some anxiety about possible delays in discharge from hospital, particularly for elderly patients, but no real expectation of disaster.

There is, however, an important exception to this rather cautious view of the changes, and an encouraging one for the future. Those I spoke to in social services probably have the clearest understanding of the changes as they are evolving and they were the most enthusiastic. The social worker who has real experience of the new system, and who in a pilot project has the flexibility and funds to operate it, believes that the changes can greatly benefit users and carers.

1 *The all-Wales mental handicap strategy: framework for development from April 1993.* Cardiff: Welsh Office, 1992.
2 *Mental illness services: a strategy for Wales.* Cardiff: Welsh Office, 1989.
3 *Caring for people in Gwent: social care plan April 1992-March 1995.* Newport: Gwent County Council, 1992.
4 Secretary of State for Health. *The health of the nation: a strategy for health in England.* London: HMSO, 1992. (Cm 1986.)
5 *Pathfinder strategies for health.* Newport: Gwent Health and Gwent Family Health Services Authority, 1991.
6 Pathy MSJ, Bayer A, Harding K, Dibble A. Randomised trial of case finding and surveillance of elderly people at home. *Lancet* 1992;**340**:890-3.

Bassetlaw: "The planning process has not been easy"

TRISH GROVES

Bassetlaw is a mainly rural council district in Nottinghamshire, just north of Robin Hood's Sherwood Forest. Its population of 105 000 is concentrated in two market towns, Worksop—known as the gateway to the Dukeries because the wooded hills nearby once belonged to great ducal estates—and Retford, one of the oldest chartered boroughs in the country.

Unemployment among Bassetlaw's men last year was just less than England's overall rate of 9·7%. This could increase, however, if Retford's local coal mine, Bevercotes Colliery, closes. Its almost immediate closure was announced and then retracted in autumn 1992, and its 600 or so employees have been waiting to hear how long the reprieve will last. Manton Colliery, near Worksop, is scheduled to stay open but is no longer recruiting staff to replace those who leave or retire.

In the population census for 1991 nearly one in seven of Bassetlaw's residents said that they had long term illnesses, health problems, or handicaps that limited their daily activities or work. How many of them need but do not receive community care is not known. From April, however, there will be closer cooperation among the various statutory and voluntary services that arrange and provide care and, in the long run, this might lead to more efficient recognition of ill or disabled people who need help with daily life.[1] I visited Bassetlaw last month to see how its community care services work now and how they are set to change.

Making plans for Bassetlaw

Joint planning

Bassetlaw's community care services will change along with those for the whole of the county of Nottinghamshire. Despite goodwill and a developing sense of partnership among social services, health authorities, the family health services authority, and the voluntary sector, the planning process has not been easy. The main reasons are broadly political.

Firstly, the county's health authorities and councils do not share the same boundaries, and the existing boundaries are changing. The district health authority of Bassetlaw, for example, merged with that in Central Nottingham last year to form a much larger North Notts district, and this year the nationwide reorganisation of council boundaries will reach Nottinghamshire. Secondly, some people I spoke to thought that local planning had been slowed by uncertainty about last year's general election and the possibility that a Labour government might have diluted or delayed the community care reforms.

Implementing the county's plans will not be easy, either, because of underfunding. The money being transferred from the Department of Social Security to Nottinghamshire for buying residential care will fall short of the amount needed by almost a fifth.

Assessment and care management

The government's guidance on assessment and care management is loose enough to allow different interpretations. In Nottinghamshire the social services departments will use teams rather than individual care managers to assess people and arrange packages of care. To test the new procedures, however, county hall decided to spend some of last year's specific grant for mental illness on four new care managers.

In Bassetlaw the care manager for mental health is on maternity leave and the existing social work team is trying out the new procedures. Joy Gibson, senior social worker for mental health, told me that about 50 people with complex needs are being helped in this way. Each gets a written care plan and a named key worker. When the plan is up and running and all the identified needs for care are being met, the managing team backs away and performs only intermittent reviews. The system is too new for any conclusions to be drawn yet, but one problem has developed already. The social work and psychiatric teams have different criteria for deciding who needs such

BASSETLAW: "THE PLANNING PROCESS HAS NOT BEEN EASY"

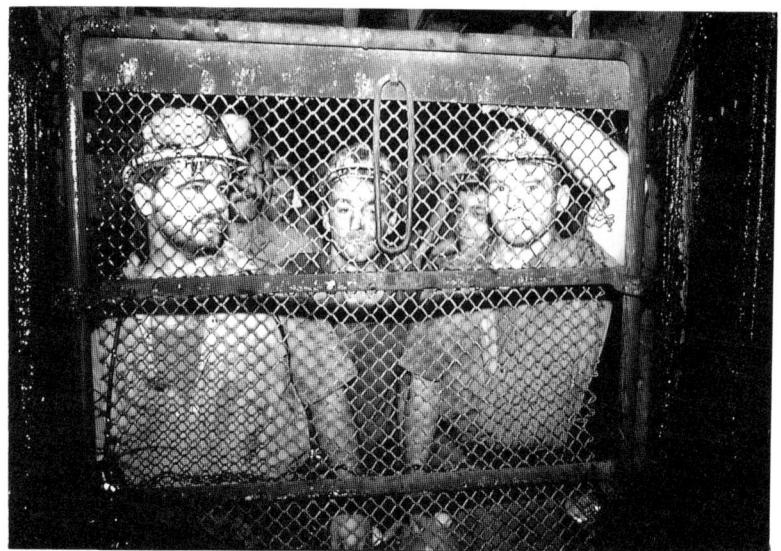

When employment is under threat the entire community feels the stress

intensive community care. The psychiatric team puts the number of local mentally ill people with complex needs at around 150, three times the social work team's estimate. Although this disparity reflects the real world of budget limits, it could scupper the care programmes that the psychiatry department is meant to set up for seriously mentally ill patients and make planning for discharge more difficult.

Discharge from hospital

An all too common kind of crisis for community and primary care teams is that a vulnerable patient is suddenly discharged from hospital on a Friday afternoon without any formal referral or plan for aftercare. To avoid this kind of disaster, health authorities in England and Wales will soon have to ensure that proper preparations for community care are made before inpatients who need such care are discharged. The down side, of course, is that hasty discharges often result from shortage of beds and thus the new procedures will probably block beds.

Geriatrics beds are those most likely to be blocked while assessment teams explore alternatives to residential care. At present two thirds of all people admitted to Nottinghamshire's nursing homes go straight from hospital, and most are elderly. In Bassetlaw the liaison sister for elderly people, Frances Fairclough, has been seconded to look generally at community care planning and specifically at discharge procedures.

Over the past year Mrs Fairclough has piloted a scheme with one general practice on discharge planning. All patients from that practice who have been admitted to any department of Bassetlaw Hospital (except the units of psychiatry and paediatrics, which have their own similar systems) have been assessed on admission for their likely needs on discharge. Using a special form, nursing staff have recorded and updated these needs. When a patient in the scheme is discharged a copy of the form, which also has room for the ward doctor's summary and details of any prescription, is faxed to the patient's general practitioner. So far, the scheme is working well. But other aspects of the reforms are still bothering some of Bassetlaw's general practitioners.

The GP's role

One general practitioner, who works in a large multipartner practice in Worksop, said that the community care reforms were all a bit of a mystery. Although he knew the basic principles of assessment and care management by social services, he did not know what his own role in the process might be. Feeling overloaded with routine and emergency clinical work (there are no deputising services in Bassetlaw) and with administration, he did not see how he and his colleagues could commit any extra time to assessment.

One of the district's few fundholders was concerned that he had not yet had enough information on how he will be able to buy community health services in April. "No one has told us how this will work," he said. "I presented the district health authority with a list of questions on this three months ago and I've had no reply. For instance, what will happen when we refer patients to the new community mental health team that's being set up? Referrals to community psychiatric nurses are chargeable to the fund but those to social workers are not. This could cause problems with data collection." He was also worried that social workers on the care management team would have the final say on choosing nursing care. If he wanted to refer a patient to a nursing home and the social work team recommended district nursing in the patient's own home, he would not only be overruled but also have to foot the bill for the nurse.

Tony Ruffell, chief executive of Nottinghamshire family health services authority (FHSA), told me that preliminary research in the county suggested that each general practitioner would encounter only a few such difficult decisions a year—perhaps five or six. Regarding the extension of fundholding to community health services such as district nursing and occupational therapy, he said that fundholders would have to make block contracts in the first year.

Monica Gellatly, community care coordinator for the FHSA, explained why general practitioners were feeling so much in the dark about the changes. "We couldn't start training GPs until we knew what was going to happen locally. Just describing the general principles and answering specific questions with 'we're working on it' wouldn't have been good enough." In January and February the FHSA put the record straight by sending all general practitioners in Nottinghamshire an information pack and inviting them to a range of training sessions on community care. These sessions included four evening "roadshows" of presentations and workshops, which were illustrated with real examples of how the reforms will be handled locally. Those who attended could claim the postgraduate educational allowance.

Thus, general practitioners in Bassetlaw should soon know what kind of role they will have in assessing people for community care. To facilitate such assessments a joint working party of general practitioners and the FHSA, chaired by Professor Idris Williams from Nottingham University, is producing a standard protocol. The end result of the working party's efforts and a small pilot project in four representative practices should be a single assessment form for doctors to complete. The Department of Health has not decided yet how much general practitioners will be paid for work that exceeds their contractual obligations, such as attending care management meetings and performing certain assessments.

Delivering care

Last year Bassetlaw's district general hospital in Worksop and its related community services became an NHS trust. According to Dr Peter Pratt, who heads the trust's community health directorate, the unit is particularly well set up to respond to the increasing emphasis on non-hospital care in the NHS. He explained that the district hospital has developed a strong sense of community service, partly because it has always had to find ways of reaching a scattered population. Staff are more willing, perhaps, than those in high profile

BASSETLAW: "THE PLANNING PROCESS HAS NOT BEEN EASY"

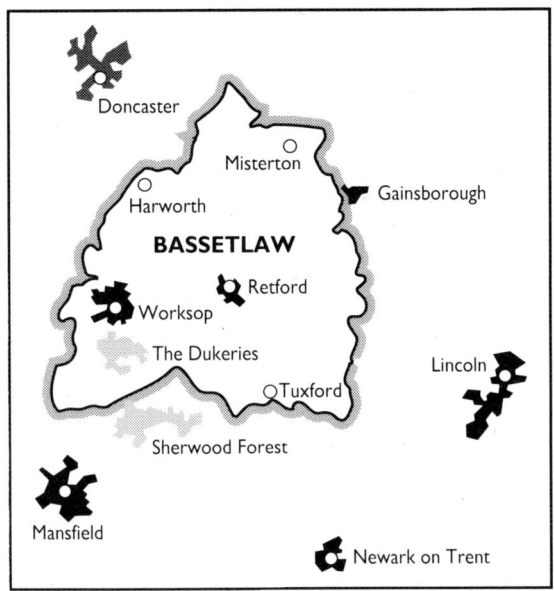

Bassetlaw's community care services have to reach a scattered, mainly rural population

academic centres to accept the idea that there will be a move away from a hospital based service.

One impending move is the closure of the last remaining ward in Worksop's old Victoria Hospital. It houses long stay elderly patients who will move to a new community unit in 1993 if all goes to plan. Residential care for elderly people is, perhaps, the hottest issue for local planners: of all the districts in the Trent health region, Bassetlaw has the fastest growing population of people over 85. This is mainly because many of the district's relatively cheap large houses have become part III and nursing homes, offering about 300 places in the private sector and around 150 run by social services.

Elderly people

Of Bassetlaw's 18 000 pensioners, more than 2500 live alone. Fewer than half of the district's households that include a pensioner have a car. It is easy to understand, therefore, that social isolation is a particular problem for local elderly people. Joan Bower of the voluntary organisation Age Concern told me how her local branch takes services to its clients, rather than making them travel. Volunteers run

17 luncheon clubs and three coffee bars around Bassetlaw, many of them in small outlying villages. Last year they served some 19 000 council subsidised meals to elderly people. Both Age Concern and the social services department have set up befriending schemes, sending volunteers or care assistants to spend time with elderly people at home and often giving carers a break.

In addition to practical help, some carers looking after elderly relatives and neighbours may need emotional support. Lynne Moody, nursing sister in Bassetlaw's day hospital for elderly people, runs an informal support group for carers. Because the day unit concentrates on rehabilitation and has a fairly fast turnover none of the eight people who come to talk over tea or coffee has a relative attending the day hospital at the moment. Mrs Moody would like to advertise the group more widely and would be happy to invite former carers whose elderly charges have died or gone into residential homes. She has found that the decision to choose residential care can cause just as much bereavement and guilt as can death.

There is no separate department of geriatric medicine in Bassetlaw. All four physicians admit elderly patients into the district hospital's general medical beds. The medical teams already hold multi-disciplinary case conferences to plan continuing care for elderly patients with complex needs. After April they intend to use the standard discharge procedures that have already been piloted with one general practice, as mentioned above. Dr M M Muthiah, consultant physician, told me that existing good relations with social services and other disciplines should ensure a smooth transition to the new style of community care. He was worried, however, that adherence to the new pre-discharge procedures might block acute medical beds unless care management teams were funded adequately and could respond quickly.

Elderly people with mental illnesses get psychiatric care from the department of psychogeriatrics at Bassetlaw Hospital. Those with dementia may attend the day hospital for the elderly one day a week and may be supported in the community by one of two specialist psychiatric nurses. Penny Peysner, senior social worker at Bassetlaw Hospital, told me that the district had planned to open a special day centre for elderly mentally ill people at a social services residential home, using the mental illness specific grant. That home, however, has just been closed down as part of a refurbishment programme. She hopes that the money will be used instead to improve day facilities for this group at other homes or to set up a mobile day unit.

People with mental health difficulties

"We have been bashing out plans for care management and for better discharge procedures, and on paper we can offer community care very well," said Jim Walker, acting director of Bassetlaw trust's mental health services. "There will be even better scope for teamwork. I don't think we could ever have made *Caring for People* work when the CPNs were here in the hospital and the social workers were 10 miles away in Retford." From April social workers, the CPNs—community psychiatric nurses—and a psychologist should be working together in a new community mental health resource centre in the middle of Worksop. The centre will be housed in doctors' old residences and Joy Gibson, senior social worker for mental health, will head the team.

But Jim Walker told me that, despite these good developments, he was worried that the new system for community care might be underresourced. All the services for mental health seemed to be at full stretch already, he said. The expected shortfall in social services funding for community care had already led to tightening of the criteria that social workers will use to decide who is eligible for care management, and patients with moderate needs for care might lose out altogether. In addition, the hospital's psychiatric unit could not cope with bed blocking: occupancy often reaches 90% in spring and autumn, leaving inadequate space for emergency admissions.

The recommendations of the Reed report, that mentally ill offenders should be cared for by local NHS psychiatric services, could tip the balance even more, said Jim Walker. Ranby prison, midway between Worksop and Retford, would turn to Bassetlaw Hospital for its prisoners' psychiatric care. This could add considerably to the existing demand to rehabilitate patients from Rampton special hospital, which also lies within Bassetlaw.

Patients with severe mental illness who need long term rehabilitation are relatively well served in Bassetlaw. Worksop has two NHS run and fully staffed hostels in the hospital grounds and a 16 bedded hostel run by the charity Turning Point. I visited these facilities two years ago, when the new community care legislation was being set up.[2] Last month Trevor Goodall, team leader of the Turning Point project, told me, "Bits of information on the community care changes are filtering through to us from social services, and we think that we will be involved in the assessment process. Our existing residents will continue to get social security funding for their rent and we assume that we will still get grants from the health authority and social services for our running costs. We hope the changes won't alter things too much."

Concentrating the resources for community care on people with severe mental illnesses makes sense. Other people with less florid but equally chronic mental health problems, however, could find it much harder in future to get help from the busy statutory services. I spoke to Jean Collis, coordinator of Bassetlaw MIND (the local branch of the national association for mental health), who was worried that people with chronic depression and anxiety would have to rely increasingly on voluntary organisations for help. The local support groups and befriending schemes that MIND was running two years ago[2] are expanding all the time, and a new advocacy service to help people with mental health problems deal with lawyers, the courts, doctors, and other professionals is taking off. But Mrs Collis has found raising funds for these services particularly hard in the past year.

People with learning disabilities

Schemes for befriending and advocacy are also available for Bassetlaw residents with learning disabilities. These are run by both social services care assistants and volunteers. The community mental handicap team (a title it retains, although its members do not describe their clients as handicapped) has more than 10 years' experience of providing such innovative care to a mainly rural and home based population. A survey in 1989 showed that the team knew of 350 local people with severe learning disabilities, of whom 217 lived with their families and 38 lived with single carers.

Bill Barker, senior social worker, explained that the team had served children as well as adults with learning disabilities until last year. Under the terms of the Children Act, however, responsibility for helping these children now lies with the social services child care team. Although this transfer of responsibility makes sense in many ways, it hampers continuity of care for a group of people with long term needs. Such continuity might also suffer under the new legislation on community care.

"Many families are struggling on, perhaps because they don't want to consider residential care or because the right sort of care isn't available," said Bill Barker. "Helping people with learning disabilities and their families is often a very gradual process. I'm worried that the changes to community care might, paradoxically, spoil this long term relationship. If our priority is to target help at those with most need and to back away when those needs are met, our contacts with families could become simply box-ticking sessions, and it would be harder to get to know them."

People with learning disabilities who need residential care in Bassetlaw can go to one of four staffed homes which were set up partly by the health authority and are run by the Mencap Homes Foundation. From April the rent of new residents will be funded by the council's community care budget. Karen Sands, of the foundation, said that she had no particular worries about the changes in the short term. She wondered, however, whether the philosophy of matching services closely to needs might eventually mean that existing residents who were relatively independent might be thought unsuitable for Mencap's homes. "We tell our residents that this is their home, and we do not always expect people to move on," she explained.

Dr C L Narayana, the consultant who covers mental handicap services for the whole North Notts district, works two sessions a week in Bassetlaw. He told me that he too had no particular worries about community care and that the provision of residential care was very good. The only shortfall, he said, was of facilities for patients with very difficult and challenging behaviour. Balderton Hospital in Newark, the old mental handicap hospital for the county, is set to close this year, and Bassetlaw's small inpatient unit cannot provide long term intensive care.

People with physical disabilities

Community social services for people with sensory and physical disabilities are provided from the Eastgate Centre in Worksop. A team of social workers and support staff offers advice and practical help and the day centre provides social contact for about 100 people a day. Molly Allen, the disability team manager, explained how the service is moving away from the traditional model of care. The team's philosophy is to encourage disabled people to help themselves and each other, particularly by running parts of the centre themselves. Block funding comes from social services, and Mrs Allen does not foresee any change after April.

Community health services for people with disabilities, such as physiotherapy and occupational therapy, are provided by Bassetlaw trust. Like others I spoke to, Dr Peter Pratt aims to send as many services as possible from his community health services directorate in Retford Hospital to the rural areas of the district. For example, two new mobile units are now taking chiropody and dentistry to the villages. As a member of Nottinghamshire's interagency planning team, Dr Pratt has been involved in setting up community care for the county. He said that he was generally optimistic about the plans and thought that Bassetlaw's combined hospital and community trust was well set up to implement them, not least because the trust has good information systems.

Conclusions

Bassetlaw particularly needs good community care because many of the people who most need help live outside the towns and lack easy access to hospitals and town halls. The district's services seem to reflect this need well already, perhaps because Bassetlaw does not have a teaching hospital to concentrate NHS resources or a city to exhaust social services. Most importantly, the people who will have to implement the community care reforms seem to share the same vision and, despite certain reservations, the same enthusiasm.

1 Secretaries of State for Health, Social Security, Wales, and Scotland. *Caring for people: community care in the next decade and beyond.* London: HMSO, 1989. (Cm 849.)
2 Groves T. After the asylums: the local picture. *BMJ* 1990;**300**:1128-30.

Northern Ireland: building on integrated services

ALISON TONKS

The community care reforms depend on close cooperation between health and social services. Sceptics have suggested that differences in the training and philosophy of those in the two services might lead to difficult culture clashes. In Northern Ireland, however, health and social services have been integrated for 20 years and this may give the province a head start in coping with the reforms.

Until 1990 the two branches had separate professional lines of management, but since then services have been united all the way down from administrators in the Department of Health and Social Services to the professionals providing care. Local authorities, which have responsibility for social services in the rest of the United Kingdom, do exist in Ulster, but they deal exclusively with municipal and environmental health tasks such as emptying dustbins and cleaning the streets.

The organisational hierarchy has only three tiers. At the top is the Department of Health and Social Services. Below this are the province's four health and social services boards: northern, southern, eastern, and western. The boards are split up further into units of management: administrative areas that contain varying numbers of hospitals, health centres, and other providers of community services. The Eastern Health and Social Services Board has nine units of management. Four of them are community units, although within this, they may manage a small acute hospital. Some hospitals, such as the Belfast City Hospital, are units of management on their own.

Planning community care with an integrated service

During a visit to Northern Ireland I spoke to Margaret Bamford, assistant director of social services at the Eastern board, and Bob Moore, the board's social services director. They both agree that integration has helped the planning of community care. Firstly, local authorities and health authorities don't have to make special efforts to get together to make plans. Secondly, the transfer of funding between health and local authorities that has proved so difficult in other parts of Britain is unnecessary in Northern Ireland. Finally, integration makes it easier for professionals and managers from each side to talk to each other and begin to bridge the cultural divide between them.

Bob Moore insisted that integration was not a panacea for the potential woes of community care. "Because of integration our units of management haven't been able to become NHS trusts. At the moment there is no legal framework allowing social services to be trusts. Our units of management will have to wait for enabling legislation to go through before they can become trusts in 1994." Margaret Bamford also added a cautionary note: "Integration is far more evident at senior management level than at the grass roots. The nearer to the patients you get, the greater the divide," she said.

Rene Boyd, retired social worker and former assistant director of social services, agreed that social workers and health workers still speak different languages. "When a social worker asks if a patient can walk she means, 'Can that patient walk well enough to go home?' When doctors talk about a patient walking they mean anything from trotting up hills to taking a few steps heavily supported by four people."

Cultural differences

The cultural and demographic differences that separate Northern Ireland from the rest of Britain work both ways for the health and social wellbeing of the people who live here. Disability in general is commoner, and the prevalence of coronary heart disease is higher. Data from Northern Ireland's Policy Planning and Research Unit show that the incidence of disability among adults is 174/1000, and that 20/1000 are severely disabled. About 17% of the total population has some form of disability.

On the other hand, the closeness of the community and strong family ties mean fewer homeless young people on the streets of

Belfast. "Young people here always have somewhere to go, either to family or friends," says Dr Raymond Shearer, a general practitioner in Crocus Street, near to the troubled centre of Belfast. "Homelessness isn't non-existent, but it is nothing like as bad as in some English cities."

A strong sense of spiritual identity and loyalty within families also means that there is a social network of support from family, friends, neighbours, and the church. Many people I spoke to mentioned the willingness of the Northern Irish to care for their elderly and disabled relatives at home, sometimes with minimal help. "I am constantly humbled by the decency of the folk out there," says Dr Shearer. "Some of the young people in particular are very generous with their time."

Planning community care in the Eastern board

The Eastern Health and Social Services Board is the biggest of the four boards. About 635 000 people live within its area; 44% of the population of Northern Ireland. It covers an area extending from North Belfast to the Mourne mountains in the south and includes most of the city of Belfast. The city is fairly small, with a population of less than 400 000, about the same as Bristol. There are only 1·5 million people living in the whole province.

Belfast's teaching hospitals and tertiary referral centres all fall within the Eastern board's remit. Until now the city attracted the largest slice of the funding cake from the Department of Health and Social Services. From 1 April 1993, however, this board's directors have to deal not only with new funding arrangements for community care but also with a considerable loss of revenue because its specialist centres and teaching hospitals will not attract any extra money. Funding will be calculated on a per capita basis for each board, regardless of the facilities available in each. The end of preferential funding for the Eastern board means that it will have to implement the community care changes with a total budget reduced by £51m.

Despite this setback to the board's finances, Bob Moore and Margaret Bamford were confident that all the operational structures needed to cope with the new arrangements would be in place by April. They both agree with the principles behind the NHS and Community Care Act 1990 and the policy paper that detailed the reforms in Northern Ireland, *People First*.[1]

Bob Moore has certain reservations about putting the theory into

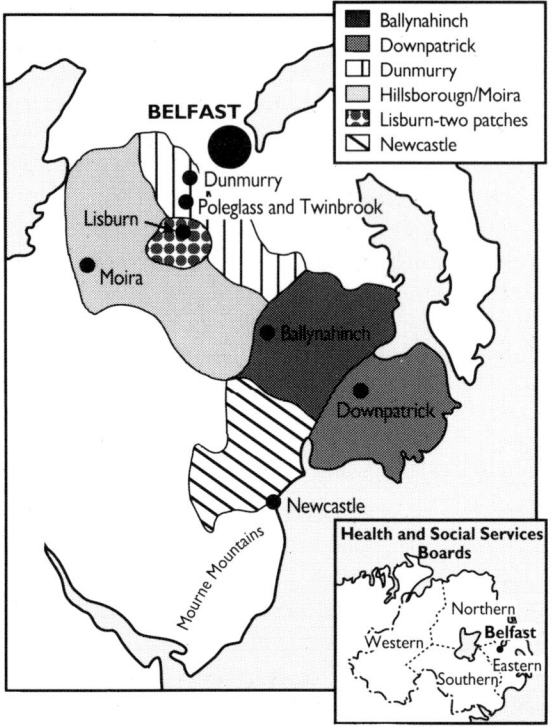

Patches in the Eastern board's Down and Lisburn unit of management. Patches are based around general practices and each has an integrated primary care team

practice. "The needs led approach is ideologically sound," he said, "but it's possible that its implementation could be paralysed because of lack of funding. The whole of Northern Ireland is getting only £4m extra to set up the new funding arrangements. I don't think it will be enough. The government is trying to get community care on the cheap and that will mean only one thing — rationing." He is also concerned that the board could end up being taken to court if the funds were not available to meet a client's assessed needs.

Margaret Bamford also has reservations. "The Department of Health and Social Services has set a target that, by 1997, fewer than 12% of the over 75s should be in institutional care. That figure at the moment stands at 16-22%. This means that if we meet the target some residential and nursing homes may well go out of business; a very grave prospect in the current gloomy economic climate."

A working group, chaired by Margaret Bamford and including representatives from the units of general management, has written a detailed draft document outlining the process of care management. The final draft will form the basis for contracts between the board and the units of management that will provide the care through their hospitals, health centres, community health services, statutory social services (for example, the provision of home helps), and residential homes for elderly people. The units of management will also be given a budget to purchase a "mixed economy" of social care from the voluntary and private sector.

Down and Lisburn unit covers half the area of the Eastern board and serves a quarter of its population. The area is diverse: some of the richest and some of the poorest people in the province come under the unit's remit. It covers the deprived areas of Poleglass and Twinbrook that spill out of west Belfast, the privileged commuter belt, and the scattered rural communities that spread out towards the Mourne mountains in the south.

Brian Dornan, an assistant unit general manager, explained that in anticipation of the changes to community care Down and Lisburn unit had been divided into "patches." Each patch is based around a general practice and has a patch team. The patch teams—or integrated care teams—include a general practitioner, community health professionals, and social workers. For example, the patch team in Dunmurry is based around a general practice with four partners. The team is made up of three district nurses, a nursing auxiliary, a midwife, two health visitors, a part time social worker, and a social work assistant.

Each of the unit's six patches has a patch manager and an assistant patch manager. One is a nurse and one a social worker. The patch arrangement was successfully piloted in Dunmurry at the beginning of 1992 and is now fully operational. Detailed plans for assessment and care management have been drawn up, so that when open access to residential and nursing homes for the elderly ends, there will be someone on the spot who knows how to get the assessment procedures going. That person will be the patch manager. Eventually, patch managers will take over the budget for care management.

Brian Dornan is highly committed to the patch model. He believes that patch teams should be well placed to cope with the biggest change—care of frail elderly people. Arrangements for other groups of disabled people are still evolving in unit wide programmes. Like everyone else at the planning end, Brian Dornan is concerned about funding. The changes will mean new employees such as accountants, who will have to be paid. Exactly how much money there will be and who will get it is yet to be worked out.

The carers

There are an estimated 210 000 carers in Northern Ireland, according to the Carers National Association. Without them current government policy would be a nonsense. They are unpaid and, as Raymond Shearer pointed out, largely uncomplaining. Bill Love, the Northern Ireland development worker for Carers National Association, is guardedly optimistic. "On paper the changes look good for carers," he said, "but as always there are funding constraints."

Patricia Jenkins has been caring for her disabled daughter for seven years. She knows all about funding constraints. Laura-Lee was 2 when she developed a spinal tumour—an ependymoma—and she is now paraplegic and dependent on a wheelchair. Caring for her is a full time job.

Mrs Jenkins' marriage has broken up because, as she puts it, "there's just no room for a marriage when you're caring for someone else all the time." She also suffers from social isolation. Laura-Lee is growing up and her mother is finding it increasingly difficult to lift her into the car to go out. Her disease is so rare that there is no local group for sufferers: support groups tend to be disease specific, and Laura-Lee cannot attend groups for sufferers of spina bifida or cerebral palsy. Local respite care facilities are unsuitable because they tend to be for children with learning disabilities, so Mrs Jenkins has not had a weekend away since Laura-Lee was born. Laura-Lee was once offered respite care in England but her mother couldn't afford the plane fare.

A home help comes in for five hours a week to help with cleaning, and a social worker visits whenever something needs sorting out. Input from the voluntary services is minimal. Housing is one of the Jenkins' biggest worries. Their small three bedroomed council house is adequate but is not designed for a wheelchair. Wheelchair bungalows are available but they don't have adequate storage space for Laura-Lee's large mobility aids. Also, moving away to the area of a new unit of management could mean losing the home help.

Mrs Jenkins is well informed and active on Laura-Lee's behalf. But she often feels embattled. "Community care is really geared towards the elderly and mentally handicapped, and rightly so, but it means with a child like mine you have to fight hard for everything," she says. "I sometimes feel I have to act like a barrister or even a spy. Professionals should listen much more to the carers themselves. Only we know what it's really like."

The good news is that situations like Mrs Jenkins' should improve as agencies become more "carer aware." To this end, 11 of Northern Ireland's 18 carers' groups and associations have formed a carers' network, representing all carers in the province. Members of the network meet four times a year to discuss problems and plan strategy. Plans include training seminars for nurses and general practitioners on the special needs of carers, a conference on community care for representatives from the church, and the compilation of a carers' directory detailing all the available support and resources for carers in Northern Ireland.

Also in the pipeline are two pilot projects—one rural, one urban—which are jointly funded by the eastern and southern boards and the Princess Royal Trust for Carers. The urban project in north Belfast involves eight diverse organisations across the voluntary and statutory sectors working together to provide coordinated help and support. Improving respite care, providing training for carers, and expanding the network of local support groups are all on the agenda.

So far, so good. Bill Love's main worry is that complex or poorly managed assessment procedures could mean that carers have to wait longer for vital help. He also fears that, because of limited cash, carers could end up paying for services like home helps and respite care or even losing services altogether.

Keeping elderly people at home

Around a fifth of people over 75 live in some form of institution in Northern Ireland. Statutory beds—those run by the health and social services boards—are in the minority. Three quarters of residential home places are privately owned, as are all nursing homes. This means that elderly people who do need a nursing home place have little choice about what sort of home they live in. This is hardly a "mixed economy" of care.

The managers, social workers, and doctors I spoke to all agree that the funding changes will have a more immediate effect on the elderly than on any other group needing community support. The patch teams in Down and Lisburn play a central role in keeping vulnerable

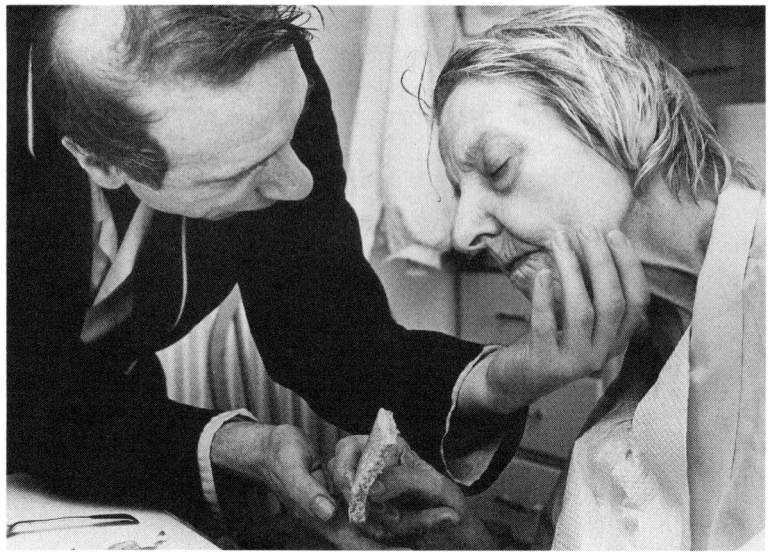
Unpaid informal carers are the heroes of the government's community care policy

elderly people at home. I visited the patch team in Dunmurry, where the model was piloted.

Denis White, one of the four general practitioner partners at the Dunmurry practice, believes that elderly people in the area get a good service from him and the other members of the team. They are all confident that every vulnerable old person in Dunmurry is known to the practice: all people over 75 are visited once a year by one of the district nurses and all patients on long term medication are seen by a general practitioner each time prescriptions need renewing.

Denis White said that, far from increasing his workload, elderly patients in their own homes called him out less often than staff in residential and nursing homes.

The vexed question of whether bed blocking will occur while patients wait for assessment before discharge from acute hospitals will gradually be answered as from April 1993 assessment before discharge is compulsory. Margaret Bamford thinks that a degree of bed blocking is almost inevitable. Mary McBrien, principal social worker for the north and west unit of management, is more optimistic. "Discharging vulnerable elderly people from acute geriatric wards shouldn't be much of a problem because geriatricians are used to multidisciplinary assessment before discharge," she said.

"The real problem will be with other specialists like orthopaedic surgeons, who are much more in the dark about assessment."

The closure of long stay geriatric beds has released funds that have been used to set up a number of community support schemes for the elderly. Money in Northern Ireland finds its way relatively easily from the closure of long stay beds into the community. The Department of Health and Social Services provides bridging loans to community projects to tide them over until the beds have been closed and the money is available.

For example, Denis White's patients have access to an intensive domiciliary support scheme. There are five such schemes currently up and running in the eastern board's area. Places on the scheme are offered to elderly people with complex needs who have had full multidisciplinary assessments. They are intended for people who would otherwise have to live in residential or nursing homes.

The Down and Lisburn scheme employs 15 full time equivalent care attendants. They visit clients as often as necessary and can help with almost anything: getting out of bed, dressing, bathing, cleaning, shopping, or lighting a fire. Schemes can also buy in other services from the voluntary or private sector. For example, Down and Lisburn's scheme sometimes uses the voluntary organisation Extra Care to provide night cover. Joe Dunne, Down and Lisburn's programme manager for the elderly, is confident that the scheme would be able to expand. Before April there were 15 places.

Services for mentally infirm elderly people

The most vulnerable group of all are the sufferers from dementia. The closure of a ward in Lisburn's long stay psychiatric hospital, Downshire, has freed money to set up a multidisciplinary dementia team based in a health centre in rural Ballynahinch. The team has a manager, a consultant psychogeriatrician, two community psychiatric nurses, two social workers, and an occupational therapist. The team takes referrals from anywhere in the Down and Lisburn unit of management, and from anyone. Friends, relatives, general practitioners, geriatricians, or worried home helps can pick up the phone and ask for help or advice.

The project has been running for five months. It is purpose built for the government's community care policy: easily accessible, flexible, carer friendly, and keen to use as many different agencies as possible. They are already busy. One of the community psychiatric nurses has a case load of 60 clients and expects more referrals when care management gets under way.

Community schemes like these are tangible evidence that, with adequate funding and collaboration between health and social services, community care policy can really progress. There seems to be less danger in Northern Ireland than in the rest of the United Kingdom that vulnerable elderly people will get caught in the crossfire between health and social service authorities arguing over who funds what.

Chronic mental illness in younger people

Downshire Hospital is one of six long stay psychiatric hospitals in the province. The process of settling inpatients in the community is well under way. An integrated mental health programme and the availability of bridging finance has helped the resettlement process. Anyone discharged from the hospital has a care plan and a key worker, usually a community psychiatric nurse or a social worker. The key worker meets with the patient's psychiatrist weekly after discharge, which means that patients are very rarely lost to follow up.

Rosemary Simpson, Down and Lisburn's programme manager for mental health, explained that a recent survey identified all but one of the patients who had been discharged from Downshire Hospital over the past 10 years. Rosemary Simpson does not anticipate any major upheavals and expects the programme to carry on as before. They have plans to build a small "village" of houses for discharged patients within the grounds of the hospital.

Services for people with learning disabilities

Muckamore Abbey is the Eastern Health and Social Services Board's hospital for people with learning disabilities. The biggest of three such hospitals in the province, it was built in the 1950s and over the years has had varying numbers of inpatients. Dr Caroline Marriot, a consultant psychiatrist based at the hospital, estimates that there are currently about 500 inpatients. The hospital has an active resettlement programme. Since 1987 over 200 inpatients have been discharged.

Historically, says Dr Marriot, Northern Ireland has always had a more emancipated policy for people with learning disabilities than have other parts of Great Britain. In the 1940s the special care service

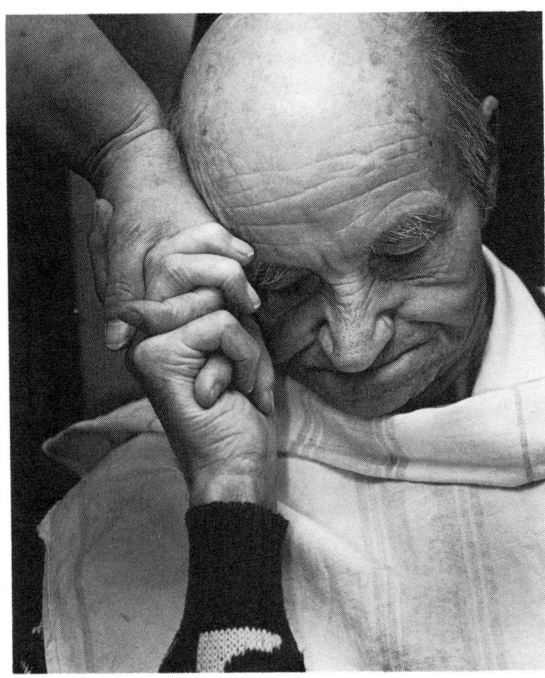

The funding changes in April will affect vulnerable elderly people more than any other group

for people with learning disabilities began. Among other things, the service established a register for the whole province. By the 1960s hostels in the community were already looking after less disabled people, so care in the community is very much the tradition here.

Dr Marriot estimates that over 70% of adults and children with learning disabilities are looked after at home. If a child is born with a learning disability and the parents are unable to cope then the baby stays in hospital until a foster family can be found.

For people needing care away from home there are a variety of different residential services. Most of the inpatients discharged from Muckamore Abbey in the past three years have gone to privately owned nursing homes. So called "core and cluster" facilities are available for less disabled people. For example, Hillhall Home in Lisburn is a modern terrace of houses which has accommodation for 16 people. This core unit is staffed but includes a three bedroomed self contained house for semi-independent living. Another 11 people live independently on the same housing estate but with support from residential home staff close by.

"Most of the community services have always been social services led," said Dr Marriot, "but, because of our integrated health and social services, there is close contact with the paramedical professions like clinical psychologists, community psychiatric nurses, and speech therapists. In theory it should be easy to access these services but in practice it's much more difficult. We have over 100 patients still in Muckamore Abbey who could leave tomorrow if the facilities were there for them to go to."

Multidisciplinary assessment and care plans are not new ideas to professionals working with people with learning disabilities. Caroline Marriot believes that their best practice fits in largely with government policy on community care. She is unsure what to expect from the implementation of care management.

Conclusion

Everyone I spoke to was completely committed to the principles laid down in the NHS and Community Care Act. Many of the managers were optimistic, whereas the providers—doctors in particular—were uncertain about exactly what was going to happen.

The amount of funding was a recurring theme and rationing came up in almost every conversation. Nevertheless, the Eastern board, at least, seems to have a solid foundation for the changes. Interdisciplinary teams are well established, managers and professionals seem to get on well, and nobody is short of ideas for what to do with any additional funding.

[1] Secretary of State for Northern Ireland. *People first: community care in Northern Ireland in the 1990s*. London: HMSO, 1990.

Newcastle: "If it doesn't work here, it can't work anywhere"

JANE SMITH

Newcastle upon Tyne, a city of 273 000 people and regional capital of the north east, starts off with several advantages for community care.[1] Some are structural —the health authority, family health services authority, and local authority are coterminous—while others stem from tradition and a strong sense of community. Despite the familiar fears about the implementation of community care—not enough money, buck passing, and bed blocking—I was struck by the optimism of social services staff. Even so, there's a clear split between the planners and the practitioners: the former see the new framework as strengthening existing good professional relationships; the practitioners, in the health service particularly, fear it as a layer of bureaucracy that may undermine those relationships.

Longstanding good relationships

Newcastle's Labour council has long had a policy of supporting its community—a policy that has informed many aspects of city life. Thus the underground transport system, the Metro, was built with disabled people in mind and council residential homes buy all their supplies locally, to support their communities. The council spends heavily on social services, partly as a general policy and partly to provide targeted services to vulnerable groups. Brian Roycroft, director of social services, is clearly proud of the standards of city provision and its responsiveness to users and carers.

Roycroft also claims—and many in the health authority agree with him—that relationships between the social services department and

NEWCASTLE: "IF IT DOESN'T WORK HERE, IT CAN'T WORK ANYWHERE"

the health authority, both managerially and professionally, have long been good and have helped underpin a high level of community care.[2] Hence his belief that if community care can't work in Newcastle "it can't work anywhere."

Implementing community care

Possibly because of this widespread feeling that relationships between health and social services were good, planning for April 1993 got left behind, and the city has spent the past few months frantically catching up. "If you had asked me a year ago," said Roycroft, "I'd have said everything was going wonderfully well—but then it all fell apart." The main problem was rate capping for the city council, which meant that the social services department had to save £4m and lose 400 staff. Homes for the elderly were shut, and formerly nominal charges increased and extended. Three of the four people on the community care implementation team left. At the same time the chairman and chief executive of the Newcastle Health Authority left amid acrimony about restructuring within the Northern region.

Realising that things were getting behind, Roycroft pulled together a policy group consisting of himself, Gary Smith, and Clare Dodgson (chief executives of the health authority and the family health services authority). Soon afterwards the chairman of the local medical committee, Dr Frankie Walters, joined the group—a move that many in Newcastle think important both symbolically and practically.

The community care plan

The core work on client groups for the 1993 community care plan is being done by the six joint care planning teams (covering aging, physical disability, learning difficulties, mental health, HIV/AIDS, and drug and alcohol problems). These have representatives of the independent sector, users and carers, ethnic minorities, and the housing department as well as social services, family health services authorities, and health authority members. Although the teams have an important role in constructing the plan, they have tended to be marginalised because they control few resources. As John Harvey, director of public health, put it, many of the teams take a very global view for their client group, consult widely, come up with good ideas, and are responsive to users, but their influence is tiny. "They have become forums for airing aspirations."

NEWCASTLE: "IF IT DOESN'T WORK HERE, IT CAN'T WORK ANYWHERE"

Harvey would like to see them bound more closely into the decision making process. As an example he cites a review that the health authority and the mental health trust have just completed of their mental health strategy, using the planning team as an important part of the consultation mechanism. One of the recommendations is that the planning team should implement the review by analysing different ways of providing particular services—crisis intervention, for example—and making recommendations to the purchasing authority.

The purchaser-provider split

To implement a purchaser-provider split within Newcastle social services department, the plan is to let the fieldwork section, based in area social work teams, act as purchasers and the residential and day

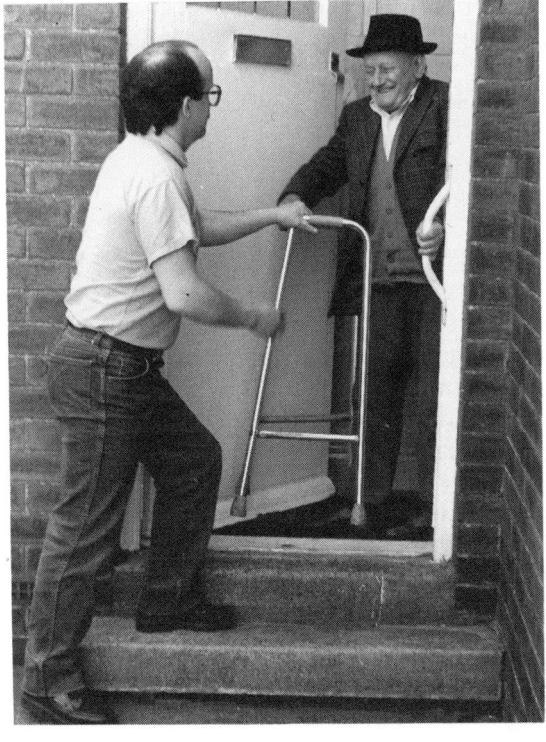

The "real backbone" of Newcastle's social services: home care . . .

care section (which includes home care) to act as providers. Few people in the department see this split as being very real at the moment, particularly as it will be some time before budgets are devolved. Roycroft doesn't particularly like the idea; he thinks assessment and provision go together for individuals—a view shared by most of his social workers.

Meanwhile the problem for the health service is that although the health authority sits on the policy group and is a coauthor of the community care plan, the work gets done—and the problems arise—in provider units. Both Gary Smith and Barry Dowdeswell, chief executive of the Royal Victoria Infirmary, Newcastle's oldest teaching hospital, agreed that the acute hospitals had only just woken up to community care. Only now are they starting to organise training for their staff. As a result, said Dowdeswell, they had realised how lucky they were with their hospital social workers: "The hospital teams have been very well protected within social services."

Nevertheless, there are fears. Roycroft and Smith worry about perverse incentives: the fact that hospital treatment costs nothing, while people have to pay for the home care that will keep them out of hospital. Dowdeswell worries about meeting contract commitments and the costs of having a geriatrician concerned in all complex assessments in elderly people. Doctors and nurses worry about bed blocking.

Within the hospital

Nurses at the infirmary have just been praised by the Audit Commission for their work on discharge planning, and a group of sisters in the orthopaedic unit confirmed that they had long taken this seriously. They discuss any problem cases with their hospital social worker each week; occupational therapists routinely make home visits before discharge; and if minor adaptations are needed a hospital technician will do them. Nevertheless, there are delays in discharge at the moment, often caused by silly things like a lack of commodes, and the nurses worry that if everything has to be in place before discharge then there will be more delays. But the blame is always with the system, not the individuals: "We're lucky with our social worker—she works wonders," said one of the sisters.

The strongest criticism I heard came from Dr Alistair Brewis, consultant chest physician and medical director of the Royal Victoria Infirmary. Not realising that the documents on discharge and assessment had been produced in a hurry to meet the government's suddenly imposed deadline of 31 December, he criticised the two weeks he had been given to consult his 200 consultant colleagues. "The act is all about communications—but here's a bad way of communicating at the outset." He found it difficult to get consultants interested in community care because it was only one on a long list of issues. Terry Sangwin, the nurse manager for the medical unit, thought staff in the hospital still needed much more information about what would happen, and she feared the planners didn't realise the impact community care might have on acute hospitals. Both she and Dr Brewis were also concerned about the many patients on their wards who came from outside Newcastle: they knew even less about the arrangements for community care within those districts.

Jackie Marston, manager of the hospital social workers, was still negotiating funding for social work links with these surrounding districts when I met her and some of her team at the hospital. They were very positive about community care and saw it as natural development of their work. Marston explained that hospital social workers had negotiated their role in discharge in the 1970s, when the Freeman Hospital had been built—"discharges don't happen without social services input"—and had then spread the same working practices to Newcastle's other two acute hospitals.

They were very aware of the fears about bed blocking. Indeed, they had just finished a three month study, half funded by the hospital "at a time when it didn't have a penny" to assess bed blocking on one medical/geriatric ward that had particular problems. The delays were caused mainly by patients waiting for long term care (because private provision hadn't kept up with demand). As a result Anne Wilson, the ward's social worker, is now funded half by the hospital to work at the Sanderson rehabilitation centre to liaise with community social workers and families.

Anne Wilson and her colleagues were as concerned as anyone that assessments are done promptly. "Not delaying assessment and placement is important to the user and family—it maintains their confidence." They too mentioned things like delays in supplying commodes that currently kept patients waiting. All these examples, they thought, simply highlighted the need for better coordination.

Indeed, Kate Weightman, programme director at the community health unit, thought that the planning envisaged by the community care plan would actually speed throughput by instilling the need to plan discharge from the outset of a hospital episode—and before when

NEWCASTLE: "IF IT DOESN'T WORK HERE, IT CAN'T WORK ANYWHERE"

possible. Her unit is already used to joint working with social services. It manages the joint inspection unit for nursing and residential homes and runs the joint loan equipment service (the one that never has enough commodes). She is also running awareness training in community care, which brings together community health staff, general practice nurses, and social workers, and her district nurses already provide some joint training for their own auxiliaries and social service home carers.

Assessment

The fear about bed blocking is acknowledged in Newcastle's assessment procedures, which speak repeatedly about the need not to delay discharge. Three levels of assessment are envisaged, and most people think that only the last of these—a complex assessment—will be new. The first level is simply to provide people with information on services—through hospitals, general practitioners' surgeries, social services offices, and public libraries. Anyone can then request an initial assessment of needs, which will be provided if the person falls into one of the client groups (elderly; mentally ill; with learning

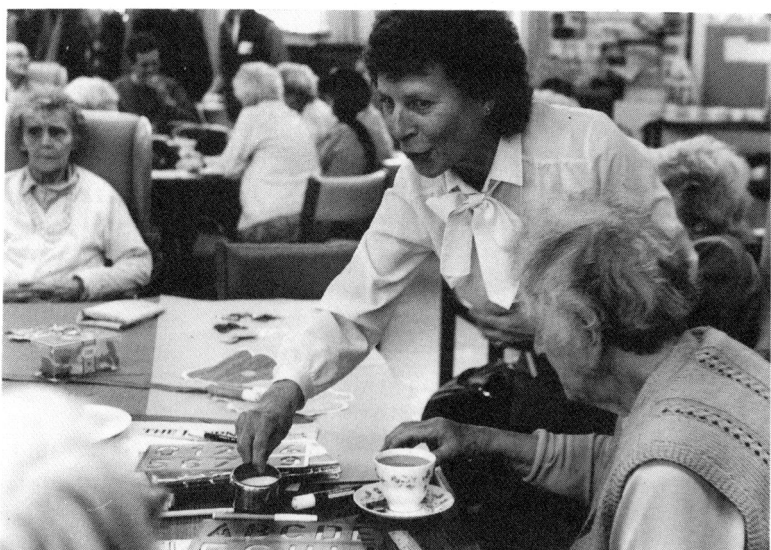

... and day care

disabilities; with physical or sensory disability or chronic illness; with drug or alcohol problems; or at risk of infection with HIV) and is experiencing difficulty with daily living.

Carolyn Stephenson, principal assistant (community care) in the social services department, doesn't think any of this is different from what staff do already. People may, for example, be referred by general practitioners, who would be expected to provide any relevant information. In future any referrer will have to provide an agreed minimum data set. Moreover, "if a person has been assessed by a general practitioner or a nurse for health reasons and they have identified social needs at the same time then we are committed to accepting that assessment," said Stephenson. She said that some social workers were uneasy about that, and she agreed that it involved trust, but it was also to avoid abandoning the problem to someone else. What is also new, she emphasised, is that the assessment is of a need, not for a particular service. It will then be up to a care manager to decide on the level of service.

This will probably involve a social worker in an area team putting together a package that might consist of a few hours of home care, a couple of days of day care, and night sitting for one night. "Probably these people don't need a formal care manager, though someone will be responsible for them," says Stephenson.

The impact of the new legislation will be felt most for people who have complex needs identified as a result of a comprehensive assessment. The key criteria are that a person has a range of needs that cannot be met by one agency alone and his or her ability to live independently is in jeopardy. This is the level where care managers will come into their own, thinks Stephenson. They need not always be social workers, and indeed, there is one care management pilot going on in the city that has a district nurse as a care manager. Here too, eventually, is where there will be budgets for care.

Budgets and services

But what will those budgets buy? Before the allocations were known the social services department had worked out that ideally it would need £5.75m. It has got £3.2m. Already some social services have long waiting lists because demand outstrips supply. Nevertheless, Graham Armstrong, assistant director of social services responsible for finance and administration and now leading the community care project team, is more worried about the second and

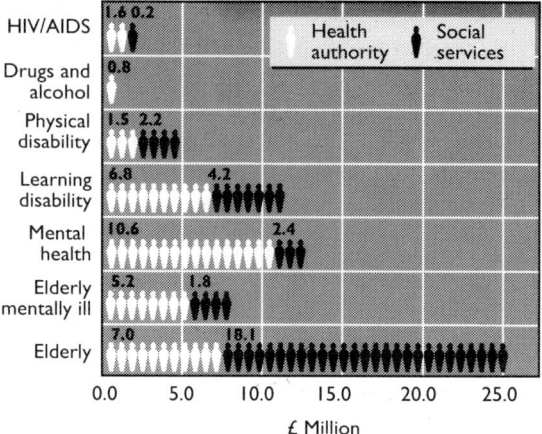

Expenditure on social and continuing health care services in Newcastle in 1991-2 by health authority and social services

third years. Ninety per cent of people in residential care in Newcastle are on income support and the average time to death or discharge in residential care is three years, so his department will be picking up the whole burden by the third year. The main shift as he sees it is that the service has become cash limited overnight. "So we have to get the eligibility criteria tied down very tight. Yet if you establish criteria for nursing and residential care you are adjusting to resources, not need."

In the first year Armstrong's concern is to go for a minimum safe agenda—"make sure clients are safe and then build on that." He has not therefore got very far with devolving budgets. From 1993 they are being allocated to area managers but not yet to care managers. This fits in with the traditionally tight control that local authority finance directors like to keep. Armstrong's other concern is that budgets should be tightly tied to the information strategy, and his department is not far advanced with that.

Another concern is to ensure that new sorts of responsive services are there to meet identified needs. As well as managing the market, the social services department is having to nurture it. Stephenson thinks that unless there are no informal carers (in which case providing continuous support at home is much more expensive than residential care) much can be done to keep even very dependent people at home. But first those services need to exist. A night sitting service, for example, needs a certain number of permanent trained staff. "So there will have to be some block contracts to provide

NEWCASTLE: "IF IT DOESN'T WORK HERE, IT CAN'T WORK ANYWHERE"

predictability for the provider," says Stephenson. Likewise, voluntary bodies need funding to enable them to bid for contracts. The department had hoped to reach flexible service agreements with many voluntary bodies, but the city's lawyers told them they either had to give grants (guaranteeing nothing in return) or set binding contracts.

Care management

Legal problems have also dogged some innovative experiments within the care management pilots the city is running. Lynn Boyle, a social worker from area 2, told how the Inland Revenue had scuppered a plan to get unemployed women to provide informal care in return for expenses and small payments. The tax authorities insisted they put the women on the payroll.

Like her boss, Boyle doesn't see why assessment and care management should be separated. She sees assessments as involving a dialogue with the client, with social workers sometimes doing therapeutic work as part of the process. She thought enforcing a distinction would simply become bureaucratic. She also told of how social workers could stimulate resources very locally. Her area has

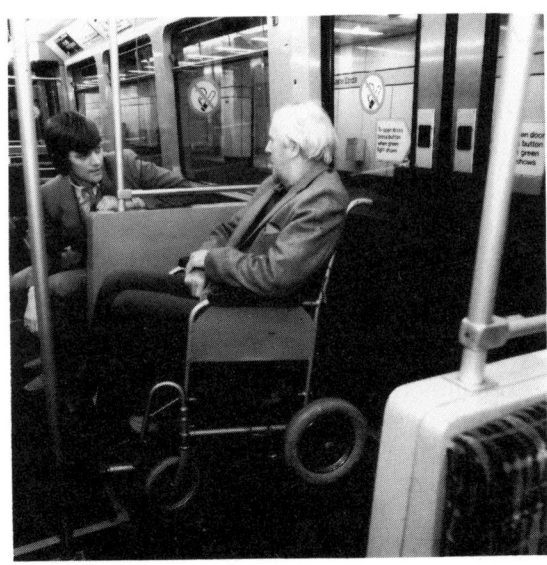

The Metro, a symbol of Newcastle's commitment to supporting people in the community

many people with learning disabilities; the community is tolerant and the housing stock suits conversion. Both the housing department and housing associations had helped with accommodation, and the social work team had started luncheon clubs and drop in centres for people with learning disabilities who did not go to day centres. They then persuaded user groups, voluntary bodies, and churches to take these services over.

Boyle also spoke of her colleagues' traditionally mixed views about general practitioners. Whether much good would came out of closer formal links between social workers and general practices very much depended on the general practitioners' attitude. "GPs don't understand what we do"—they referred inappropriate patients, and were often reluctant to pass on information. She also conceded, however, "We tend not routinely to inform GPs. There isn't a sense of coresponsibility, and we need to change that."

When the two groups do work together the outcome is better. Boyle cited a recent example of an elderly woman who was being physically abused. The doctor had helped assess the problem because she had a good relationship with her patient and had documented all her injuries. Another case in which good relationships would have helped was that of an attention seeking woman who had spent most of her life in hostels and was constantly getting struck off general practitioners' lists. "It would have been nice to have worked through the issues with the GPs and negotiated with the patient."

General practitioners

Dr Frankie Walters, chairman of the local medical committee and a general practitioner in west Newcastle, agrees with Boyle's analysis that relationships between general practitioners and social workers have not always been good. She too is optimistic that they are changing: "We are learning to talk much more openly without scoring points." As a result of her involvement in the policy group all 46 practices in Newcastle were consulted over the draft discharge and assessment arrangements and had an opportunity to influence them. The family health services authority has funded Walters's locum costs ("14 meetings in two months") and the costs of training for general practitioners and their staff, and Brian Roycroft came and spoke to well attended meetings of fundholders and non-fundholders. One thing he did was to reassure them that planning was not as far advanced as they had feared. Nevertheless, most general practitioners remained concerned about the lack of detail in the assessment and discharge documents—and were waiting to see the more detailed information promised before April 1993. They also worry that assessment procedures will raise expectations that can't be met.

Walters knows well enough not to promise to deliver for general practitioners. "The most I can do is say, 'This is what GPs are thinking.'" Also, both she and Clare Dodgson, chief executive of the family health services authority, worry that despite the well attended meetings, there are still some general practitioners who know nothing about community care. "If they don't know by 1 April, it won't be through want of trying," says Walters.

That so much effort has gone into getting general practitioners on board is a tribute to the widely held view within social services that general practitioners are not central to community care, but their capacity for throwing a spanner in the works is considerable. Yet both Clare Dodgson and John Harvey, director of public health, see beyond that.

Dodgson thinks that the debate over community care has brought out a demand among general practitioners for attached social workers, particularly among fundholders. Harvey also sees general practitioners as having a key role in the information strategy for community care. Despite the firm figures in the community care plan (see table) and social services managers' confidence that they know the

TABLE—Need in Newcastle—from 1992 community care plan

	No of people affected
Broad needs	
Continuing ill health	90 000
Age ≥ 85	4 900
Carers	30 200
Low income	52 000
Discrimination (ethnic minorities)	7 000
Vulnerable groups	
Severe learning disabilities requiring continuing care	1 000
Mental illness requiring continuing care	1 000
Homeless mentally ill	300
HIV infection	100
Alcohol or drug problems	1 400
Severe sensory or physical disability requiring care	800
Carers providing >20 h of care a week	6 500

level of need in the city, he thinks they know little. "Need is not a static concept: we need a longitudinal view and to understand how needs change." He wants to know, for example, the risk among 100 people aged over 80 of any of them needing care over the next five years—because a carer dies, they have a stroke, or they develop dementia. As part of a locality purchasing project in the east end of the city he is working with several practices to see how general practitioners can provide this sort of information.

The future

The locality purchasing project also raises questions about joint purchasing. Everyone agrees that if the service is to be seamless there are enormous benefits in having people providing care across the health—social care boundary—"one person providing bathing, bandaging, and hoovering"—and not bothering about who pays. But there are huge political difficulties with the latter. "Councillors are not going to give up their responsibility for how money is spent," says Roycroft. Themselves accountable to an electorate, councillors are sceptical about the accountability of health authorities—and about health authorities knowledge of the community: to them it's simply what happens outside hospital. Nevertheless, most of the planners in Newcastle think that the issue of joint purchasing and a wider debate about dissolving the boundary between health markets and care markets is one that the community care arrangements will increasingly force upon them.

But all that is some way off, and not confined to Newcastle. For the time being Brian Roycroft assured everyone that they wouldn't fall off a precipice on 1 April and that community care is going to work. Although Newcastle is having to run very hard to catch up with the mechanics of community care, Roycroft thinks that in terms of the spirit of the act, the city is already way ahead. "On things like consulting with patients and carers—we've been doing that for years."

1 Secretaries of State for Health, Social Security, Wales, and Scotland. *Caring for people: community care in the next decade and beyond.* London: HMSO, 1989.
2 *Partnership in action: a study of existing provision of care facilities and services for physically handicapped and frail elderly people in Newcastle.* London: Business Sciences, 1989.

PUTTING CHANGE INTO PRACTICE

Community care and the fundholder

RHIDIAN MORRIS

Background

According to the government, clearly agreed local arrangements should enable individual general practitioners to make their full contribution to the new system of community care without getting involved in extra bureaucracy.[1] From 1 April 1993 the main part of that contribution is to refer to social services those patients who seem to need social care. Many general practitioners are worried that such referrals will be complex and time consuming and will generate too much extra work. Moreover, general practitioners may also be asked to see patients specifically to help social workers' assessment procedures, and many fear that such consultations will overwork and underpay them.

General practitioner fundholders already use contracts to spell out what they expect from hospital services. From 1 April they are able to set up contracts for community health services such as district nursing and chiropody, and possibly this might be extended to social aspects of community care. For more than a year Dr Rhidian Morris and his partners in a fundholding practice in Devon piloted contracts for all aspects of community care. In this chapter Dr Morris explains how the most radical part of the pilot project—the contract for social care—was set up. He argues that the lessons on communication that came from what was essentially a fundholding project could apply also to non-fundholding practices.

The history of relations between general practitioners and social workers is generally poor. The two professions tend to be suspicious of each other, have little understanding of each other's roles, and have very different cultures. Social workers operate in teams, take measured approaches to problems, and rarely take decisions on their own. General practitioners work mainly as individuals supported by primary care teams. They have to make decisions quickly and virtually always alone. They are trained to do this and to be aware that they carry personal legal responsibility for their actions.

When plans for the NHS reforms were announced I quickly became an enthusiastic advocate of general practitioner fundholding, the purchaser-provider split, and the contract system. I had long believed that the primary health care team did not really work but that it could be made to do so by adhering to contracts. In 1991 I started negotiations to run a pilot project of community nursing contracts in my practice. I contracted from the local community unit a nursing team that would be led by general practitioners and would form a true practice based primary health care team. I approached Devon social services to develop a contract for referring patients from our practice for social care assessments.

Lack of knowledge

When I started discussions with the social services department I had an open mind about the service to be delivered. This was just as well, given my abysmal lack of knowledge about the department's range of services. I did not know whether having a contract would make much difference to the service delivered or to relationships between social workers and general practitioners. I simply wanted to see what would happen if I approached the problem with a contractor's mentality. The result was the hardest set of negotiations I have ever encountered, lasting some six months.

The social services managers were two or three years behind those in the NHS in developing contracts, although they were catching up fast. The biggest problem was that their whole philosophy and culture seemed alien. At first there was a lack of trust between us: I thought they were not trying hard enough as we went over and over the same issues; they thought I was trying to take over. I was the sole representative of the general practitioners. The social workers always worked as a team and whenever we met a roomful of people arrived. Their timescales for negotiations and those they proposed for dealing

COMMUNITY CARE AND THE FUNDHOLDER

with referrals were much longer than mine. I felt they wanted me to assess people's needs when that was their responsibility. There were even language difficulties. To them an urgent assessment meant "needs doing within two days" whereas to me it meant "needs doing immediately."

Although both sides became frustrated, it says much for the social workers' determination that they turned up to meetings and attempted to understand me. The breakthrough came when Plymouth Health Authority sent to the talks its contractor for community services, Chris Whitaker, and Devon Social Services Department sent its community care development officer, Tess Lomax. Chris was a former social worker who understood the social services negotiators and was trusted by them. Tess had a researcher's mind and an objective view.

Tess spent two days in the surgery. She watched how we worked and communicated and how messages and information were received, stored, and sent out. Then she asked me why we treated social services staff differently from everyone else. We did not write letters to them. We never recorded what information we sent them or received from

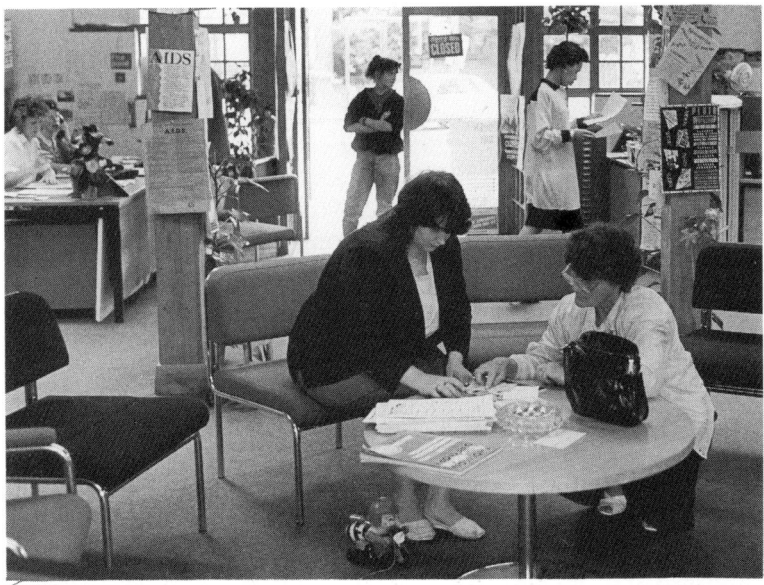

Some doctors have an abysmal lack of knowledge about the range of social services available

them. This simple observation surprised us and made us change our ways of communicating with social workers.

We decided to use the same system that we used for hospitals, making referrals to team leaders in the same way that we do to consultants. Like consultants, social services' team leaders run teams of frequently changing staff. Rapid turnover in junior staff does not disturb continuity if the working relationship is between the general practitioner and the consultant rather than the house officer. This analogy helped us to see that our previous and unsuccessful requests to have a named social worker attached to the practice had been unrealistic. At the time we had not understood why the team leader had refused this and had asked for referrals to be made directly to her.

Now that we had decided to refer to the team leader (who would be the care manager) we devised a simple referral form and agreed that all communications with and from social services would be made in writing and filed in our patients' notes. The form is very similar to that recommended recently by the BMA. Our referrals followed the same format as those to consultants and included requests for specific services when appropriate. Unlike those to consultants, however, referrals could be made by any member of the primary health care team. The contract followed fairly quickly, and on 1 January 1992 we began the pilot project.

How to do it

In the contract that we negotiated we could not alter the content of the service provided by Devon social services but we could influence the nature and speed of delivery and of communication. The contract had the basic elements of any NHS contract, plus detailed commitments for both parties (box).

The primary health care team contracted to follow set procedures for making referrals (referrers would inform patients, all referrals would include a clear statement of urgency and would be made in writing—even ones made by telephone would be followed up by written requests). Referrers also agreed to pass on relevant new information (giving advance notice to social services of cold admissions to hospital if social care might be needed on discharge, and notifying changes in circumstances of existing social services clients). Finally, leaflets and other information about social services would be displayed in the health centre waiting room.

The social services team contracted to take and act on referrals

> **Outline of contract between Ivybridge Health Centre and Devon social services**
>
> (1) Aims of contract
> (2) Duration of contract
> (3) Population to be covered (the practice list)
> (4) Brief summary of the six main acts of parliament that apply to social services and to the policy of charging clients for certain services
> (5) Grading of referrals by priority
> (6) Definitions of assessment and service provision
> (7) Procedures for quality assurance
> (8) Complaints procedures
> (9) Clear description of commitments for each party in the contract

within specified times (the office would be staffed between 9 am and 5 pm and referrals would be taken by a duty officer; urgent referrals would be dealt with within two hours, non-urgent cases would be contacted within five working days). Core assessments would be performed for all referrals, and general practitioners would be informed about assessments, services delivered, and closure of cases. Needs for social care would be identified according to the social services department's policy and budgetary constraints. Patients' needs after discharge from hospital would be monitored (separate arrangements would be made with the community health unit and hospital to assess referrals from those sources). Lastly, the social services office would display general practice leaflets and other literature.

Both parties in the contract agreed certain joint commitments, such as observing professional confidentiality, defining an out of hours service, and monitoring the contract. Monitoring included regular meetings—quarterly for the whole social services and primary health care teams and monthly for one general practitioner, the social services team leader (care manager), and the team manager of the community health unit. We also agreed to set up systems for audit (box, p 74).

All these specifications were written into the contract document. It also contained a brief description of the 30 different social care services offered, the types of patient eligible to use them, and copies of the referral form and the form used to carry out core assessments. The resulting 18 page document might seem complicated but is actually a clear and simple statement of shared commitments.

> ### Auditing the contract with social services
> We looked at the following aspects:
> - Number of referrals
> - Who is referred (age, sex, whether previously known to social services)
> - Who makes referrals
> - Urgency, quality, and complexity of referrals
> - Speed and complexity of responses, and whether made in writing
> - Problems and disabilities found on assessment
> - Service input (difference between services requested and offered, time taken to deliver services)
> - Consumer follow up
> - Contracts with primary health care team
> - Problems with contract

Monitoring the contract

As soon as we got used to our new channels of communication with the social services team the benefits of the contract became evident. Our first audit showed that in 20% of referrals the referrer had given inadequate information; the second showed that in only 7% was information inadequate. At the same time there was an increase of 15% in the complexity of referrals. Similarly, responses to us in writing within six weeks of referral rose from 25% of cases in the first audit to 60% in the second. There was also a change in source of referrals—those from district nurses rising by 34% and those from general practitioners falling by a similar amount. We have no firm data yet on whether delivery of services improved.

To explore relationships between the social services and primary health care teams the psychology department of Plymouth University carried out a questionnaire survey of attitudes. This showed that health visitors had the greatest influence on social workers. It also highlighted a complex network of contracts between the two teams and suggested the need for clear lines of communication. A member of the primary health care team has now been designated liaison officer and all messages are passed to her.

All worth it in the end

Although the contracting process was complex, it was worth while. We can now deal with the main problems that could arise in the new community care system. The Plymouth Community Trust is considering whether nurses and health visitors could order certain aspects of social care after training by the social services department. The aim is not to increase the community nurses' workload but rather to decrease time spent chasing the social work team.

Many general practitioners fear that the community care reforms will increase their own workload, too. We do not believe that general practitioners will be overburdened. In our practice, covering a population of 10 000, we make an average of 1·7 referrals a week. And we have not been asked to see any patients specifically to help social workers' assessments. We already provide medical notes for patients admitted to county council run residential homes and letters of information for those going to private care. Will there really be much change?

Conclusions

I have come through this experience with much greater understanding of social workers. I have learnt a lot from them and I recognise that we think and work in different ways. I have also learnt much from the skills of others: without Chris Whitaker and Tess Lomax we might not have succeeded in improving the way we organise community care. Though other practices may interpret and implement the community care reforms in different ways, I hope that some of the lessons we have learnt will be useful. General practitioners do not have to be fundholders to take a contracting approach to improve communication with social workers.

1 NHS Management Executive. *General practitioners and "Caring for People."* London: HMSO, 1992.

Care management and mental health

GRAHAM THORNICROFT, PAUL WARD, STEVE JAMES

Background

The community care reforms will produce a new kind of key worker who will organise and budget for packages of care: the care manager. At the time of going live in April 1993 care management is still poorly rehearsed and its performance may yet disappoint. This overview sets out the origins of case management, its transformation into care management, and the principles guiding its practice. To spell out how the concept works, plans for care management in Southwark's mental health services are described.

The roots of case management lie in social case work. Within the specialty of mental health the central coordinating function was first recognised formally in the United States by the Community Mental Health Centers Act (1963) and its 1975 amendments, which explicitly required the centres to link with other agencies providing care for long term patients. There has, however, been an increasing recognition in the United States over the past 25 years that community based services for people with long term mental illness have too often been fragmented.[1,2] Thus, methods of drawing together the components of care were developed, especially in federally funded initiatives such as the Community Support Program.[3]

The principles most often ascribed to the concept of case management are outlined in the box on p 77. Continuity of care refers both cross sectionally, to a comprehensive range of services for people with long term mental illness, and longitudinally, to emphasise the need for

> **Principles of case management**
> - Continuity of care
> - Accessible services
> - Staff-patient relationship
> - Titrating support to need
> - Facilitating independence
> - Patient advocacy
> - Advocacy for services

enduring and possibly indefinite care for a substantial proportion of this group.[4]

In practice, case management for people with long term mental illness has developed into a range of techniques that can be described along 12 different axes (box, p 78),[5] which aims to ensure that patients with long term psychiatric disorders receive consistent and continuing services for as long as they are required[6] and that services do not focus inappropriately on patients with less severe conditions.[7]

Case managers might give direct care to clients, in a model that emphasises the staff-patient relationship as the key component through which effective care is channelled, in the tradition of social case work. Brokerage models, however, give the case manager a central and more distant coordinating function without any necessary direct contact with the patient. Whichever model is used, case management offers the same range of tasks to individuals.[8-10] In Britain the concept of case management gained currency rapidly after 1985, when the House of Commons social services committee's report on community care recommended that "the government give high priority to encouraging and monitoring the developing use of keyworkers."[11] Sir Roy Griffiths took up the idea, under a different name, in 1988 in specifying that "no person should be discharged without a clear package of care devised and without being the responsibility of a named care worker."[12]

From case to care management

The 1989 white paper on community care, *Caring for People*, took the implementation of these ideas further: "Where an individual's

> **Twelve dimensions defining case management in practice**
> 1 Individual/team case management
> 2 Direct care/brokerage
> 3 Intensity of interventions
> 4 Degree of budgetary control
> 5 Health/social service function
> 6 Status of case manager
> 7 Specialisation of case manager
> 8 Staff to patient ratio
> 9 Degree of patient participation
> 10 Site of contact
> 11 Level of intervention
> 12 Target population

needs are complex or significant levels of resources are involved, the government sees considerable merit in nominating a 'case manager' to take responsibility for ensuring that the individual's needs are regularly reviewed, resources are managed effectively and that each service user has a single point of contact."[13]

The provisions of the 1990 National Health Service and Community Care Act[14] make the following statutory requirements of case managers: "Where it appears to a local authority that any person for whom they may provide or arrange for the provision of community care services may be in need of any such services, the authority (*a*) shall carry out an assessment of his needs for those services and (*b*) having regard to the results of that assessment, shall then decide whether his needs call for the provision by them of any such services."

In 1991 case management was renamed "care management" in a guidance document from the Department of Health's Social Services Inspectorate, on the grounds that the term "case" was demeaning to the individual and misleading in that it is the care, and not the person, that is being managed. At the same time, however, central guidance made it clear that the version of care management now officially sanctioned was one in which direct service provision was not included, and that a brokerage model was therefore being endorsed. This important change marked the introduction of the purchaser/provider split in social services practice, with the care manager clearly identified as a purchaser but not as a provider of services.

Implementing care management in Southwark

In Southwark the processes of assessment and care management have been planned through an interagency group comprising local authority officers, and representatives from all the health providers and purchasers and the voluntary sector. The model of assessment which has been agreed has three levels (figure). Firstly, there is a screening stage, which can take place in many community settings — for example, at social services offices, general practitioners' surgeries, and centres of voluntary organisations, or in hospital before discharge. Information is recorded on standard forms at screening and these are sent to the appropriate care management and assessment team, which is responsible for ensuring that each stage of the assessment and care management cycle is completed (box, p 80). Decisions on who needs assessment and who has priority will usually be made within the social services department, but in hospital such decisions can be made with health care staff.

The team member making the main assessment of needs for community care uses a structured form with headings covering all areas of potential need. Assessors can use an accompanying checklist to make a more detailed assessment of certain factors, allowing the resulting completed form to reflect more closely and personally the assessed person's needs. If a more detailed assessment is necessary an evaluation by a specialist can be requested, to be completed within an

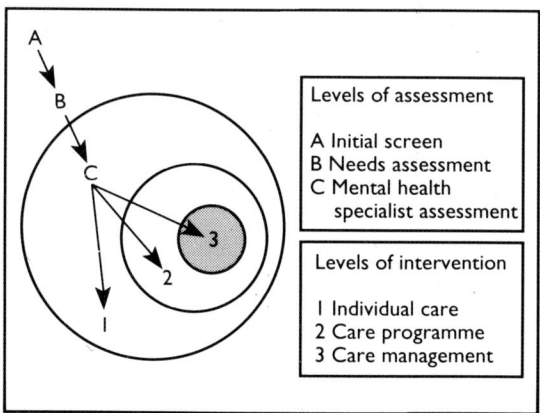

Levels of mental health assessment and treatment in care management system

CARE MANAGEMENT AND MENTAL HEALTH

> ### Stages in care management and assessment
>
> *Stage 1: Publishing information* — Making public the needs for which assistance is offered and the arrangements and resources for meeting those needs.
>
> *Stage 2: Determining the level of assessment* — Making an initial identification of need and matching the appropriate level of assessment to that need.
>
> *Stage 3: Assessing need* — Understanding individual needs, relating them to agency policies and priorities, and agreeing the objectives for any intervention.
>
> *Stage 4: Care planning* — Negotiating the most appropriate ways of achieving the objectives identified by the assessment of need and incorporating them into an individual care plan.
>
> *Stage 5: Implementing the care plan* — Securing the necessary resources or services.
>
> *Stage 6: Monitoring* — Supporting and controlling the delivery of the care plan on a continuing basis.
>
> *Stage 7: Reviewing* — Reassessing needs and the service outcomes with a view to revising the care plan at specified intervals.

agreed timescale. Throughout the process any informal carers should be consulted and should be offered their own assessments when appropriate. People being assessed are also offered an advocacy service in case they feel that they would benefit from additional support.

The model of care management planned for Southwark is mainly one of brokerage. In practice, however, social workers will still be able to offer personal help to their clients when this seems useful within the agreed care plan.

The local authority's obligation to provide services after assessment is a complex issue, with confusing messages coming from the Department of Health. Nevertheless, Southwark will provide services based on clear and publicly available eligibility criteria. Given the levels of need and the amounts of money transferred to Southwark for community care, there will probably be some unmet needs. Information on unmet needs will be collated to inform future allocation of resources.

Assessing mental health in Southwark

This model of assessment and care management will be used for all

CARE MANAGEMENT AND MENTAL HEALTH

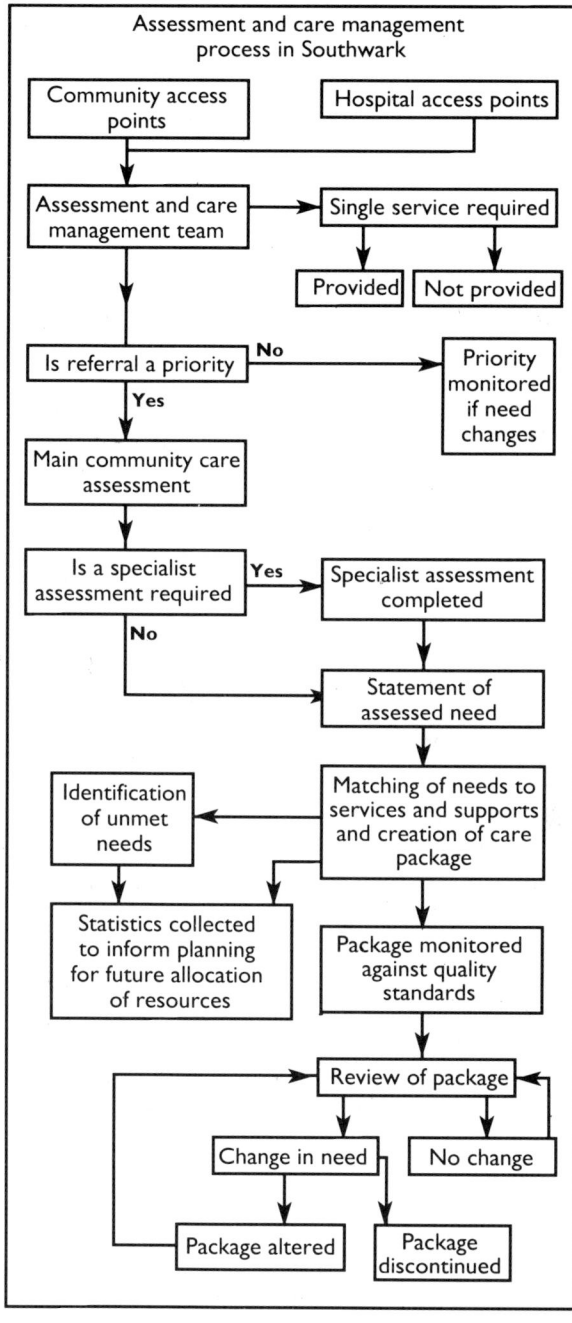

client groups in Southwark, but in the mental health services some additional features, both legislative and professional, will be incorporated into the overall structure.

Some mental health assessments are covered by separate legislation in the Mental Health Act 1983 and these will continue as at present. If such assessments result in admission to hospital the discharge policies under the NHS and Community Care Act 1990 will still apply.

Services offered to people with mental health problems after discharge from hospital may have to take into account the care programme approach,[15] the NHS and Community Care Act, and section 117 of the Mental Health Act. Southwark's model attempts to combine all the legislative requirements in one structure. It does this, for example, by defining three broad levels of service support (each with a corresponding type of service response): low (individual care), medium (care programme approach), and high (care management), where access to each of these is determined by the results of specialist mental health needs assessment.

Access to mental health services often bypasses social services departments (unlike services such as those for the elderly); thus the bulk of the initial screening will probably be undertaken by staff not working for the local authority. A high percentage of clients and patients will need complex interdisciplinary assessments. These specialist assessments may be performed by a variety of mental health professionals including social workers, psychiatrists, community psychiatric nurses, and psychologists. To make the process as uniform as possible the professionals will use standardised methods covering a range of possible problems, such as those included in the Camberwell assessment of need, which is being developed at the Institute of Psychiatry (box).

Discharge planning

Adequate discharge planning will be a key factor in introducing successfully both care management and the accompanying changes in residential care funding. The past decade has seen an increasing amount of guidance from the departments of health and social security about the need for adequate discharge policies. This guidance has become increasingly prescriptive, to the extent that the most recent document strongly reinforces the view that no discharge from hospital should occur without a clearly agreed and implemented discharge plan in place for each patient.

> **Problem areas covered by the Camberwell Assessment of Need**
>
> Accommodation
> Occupation
> Specific psychotic problems
> Psychological distress
> Information about condition and treatment
> Non-prescribed drugs
> Food and meals
> Household skills
> Self care and presentation
> Safety to self
>
> Safety to others
> Money
> Childcare
> Physical health
> Alcohol
> Basic education
> Company
> Telephone
> Public transport
> Benefits

This guidance has almost certainly improved substantially the extent and quality of discharge planning. In many cases, however, there are still important gaps between the services required and those available. This may improve as arrangements for care management are gradually introduced but for the foreseeable future plans will have to reflect a realistic view of available resources. This is particularly important if hospitals are to avoid becoming blocked with people awaiting the implementation of satisfactory discharge arrangements. When patients no longer need inpatient care but still have complex needs one of the key roles of care managers will be to facilitate rapid transfer home or to an alternative community setting.

Residential care

One of the key motives behind the current legislative changes was to find a way of limiting expenditure on residential and nursing home care, which increased from £10m in 1979 to £1bn in 1989.[13] This increase was accompanied by a substantial rise in the provision of residential and nursing home places by the private and voluntary sectors. Given the projected growth in the number of elderly people likely to need support from health and social services, this increasing cost looked set to continue.

When legislative change was being considered, attention was often drawn to the so called "perverse incentive" that saved local services money if they supported people in residential care rather than in their own homes.[12] A clear intention of the changes was to enable care managers to buy domiciliary support, rather than residential care, where this was more appropriate and less expensive. Research in Southwark, however, has suggested that only about 15% of recent referrals to residential care were inappropriate.

In April responsibility for funding residential and nursing home care will be transferred from the Department of Social Security to local authority social services departments over a phased period of four years. Thus these funds immediately become cash limited. Doubts about the adequacy of the total transfer to social services departments have already been expressed, and it is becoming clear that there may well be insufficient resources for some client groups. This is most noticeable in the case of residential care services for drug and alcohol misusers, which have a high turnover of clients. In turn, this has raised concerns about the viability of such services, and what will happen if many projects have to close while still caring for people.

This will probably be one of the flash points as the new joint arrangements for assessment and care management become established. Two other potential problems loom large. Firstly, fundholding practices may find their obligation to buy community care services a disincentive from pressing for early discharge. Secondly, patients in hospital may also avoid hasty discharge to residential or care homes if they face means tested charges. Earlier and more thorough planning may be needed before discharge, and interagency troubleshooting arrangements may have to be set up should difficulties arise.

Care management budgets

The formula dictating how social security budgets are transferred to local authorities discriminates against Southwark and most other inner city authorities in London which have few existing private and voluntary providers within their boundaries. The formula rewards authorities with large numbers of local independent providers and does not allocate resources to the authorities from which residents using that independently run care originated. Thus Southwark, which exports 70% of adults needing residential care, will not receive adequate funding to pay for future placements. This is compounded by the relatively high level of psychiatric morbidity in areas such as Southwark and by an 11% reduction in NHS funding resulting from a new weighted capitation system, which is diverting money from inner south London to Kent and Sussex.

Guidelines from the Department of Health say that 85% of the social security element of the funding transfer should be spent on residental care for elderly people with a further 5% on their day care. Clearly, this leaves the other adult groups starved of resources for residential placements. Southwark, therefore, proposes spending less—80%—of the transferred monies on services for elderly people. Of the remaining 20% of the total transfer, people with mental health problems will receive approximately 6%. This sum is inadequate and, even with rigorous prioritisation, will lead to some patients and clients having to be supported in the community when their needs could be met more adequately in residential care.

Southwark's model of care management will not devolve financial responsibility for community care to care managers. In the first year, budgets will be held by more senior staff and decision making on a day to day basis will be delegated to team managers. Very clear gatekeeping procedures and stringent setting of priorities will be needed to prevent overspending.

Care management as a purchasing function

Purchaser and provider divisions have been established in both health and social services authorities, but the splits occur at different levels. In social services departments purchasing work is oriented much more towards individuals than in the NHS, where it is oriented around services. This difference will not affect care management much in cases where social services teams are the main purchasers—for example, in services for people with learning disabilities. It is, however, much more important where the health authority is the main purchaser of community services —for example, in services for mental health, particularly in those for people with long term and severe mental illness and complex needs. For such patients decisions by care managers to commit resources will have to be integrated with the decisions about the deployment of health resources made by doctors, usually consultant community psychiatrists with specific responsibilities for discharge and aftercare under the Mental Health Act and care programme approach working in mental health multi-disciplinary teams.

Mechanisms must be set up to ensure that commissioners in both health and social services receive feedback about needs assessment.

This will be necessary if services in the NHS and those bought by care managers are to relate more closely to individual needs. This feedback will be particularly necessary in districts where care managers do not hold their own budgets.

New perverse incentives

The implementation of care management in April could rapidly illustrate how the admirable intentions of the government's community care policy might founder on the unintended consequences of more powerful forces and contradictions. Firstly, although the transfer of social security funds will allow more needs driven services, it will also cash limit expenditure. Secondly, this transfer punishes local authorities with few residential care homes and cuts off money for future expansion. Thirdly, the directive that care managers should not themselves give direct care runs counter to the core of good social work practice and creates a new corps of care administrators, thereby reducing the number of staff available to give direct care. Fourthly, no central guidance has emerged on how to coordinate, at the local level, care management,[14 16] the care programme approach,[15 17] and hospital discharge procedures, thus inviting triplication of planning effort.

Fifthly, conflicting central guidance is emerging about the statutory requirements to provide services for people whose assessments show up unmet needs, or even to inform people about the results of assessment.[18] Finally, the distinction between health and social care is proving much less clear in practice than in concept, and long running boundary disputes between agencies could erupt unless the problem is considered specifically in joint planning forums. Such joint planning is taking place now in Southwark.

Managing care management carefully

There is the ever present danger that insufficient overall funding will drown the potential benefit of the community care reforms.[19 20] And, for the current volleys of reforms to hit their targets, several extra initiatives will be required. When needs assessment information is fed into discussions on commissioning and planning it will probably highlight the need for district health authorities and local authorities (and, increasingly, general practitioner fundholders) to commission many community services jointly. Joint commissioning arrangements will allow specific gaps in service provision to be filled. Variations in joint commissioning practice between social services and health services will have to be piloted and monitored carefully. Agencies will have to agree on definitions of needs and how people with different degrees of need will be prioritised when services are rationed. The division between health and social needs can be narrowed by joint training. Agreed procedures for appeals, complaints, and arbitration should be set up for users, and for authorities in dispute. Finally, models of care management must be tracked carefully and evaluated to show whether brokerage is the hub or the rub of community care.

We are pleased to acknowledge the helpful contributions of Matt Muijen and Peter Ryan of Research and Development for Psychiatry and of Geraldine Strathdee of the Maudsley Hospital in preparing this paper.

1 Braun P, Kochansky G, Shapiro R, Greenberg S, Gudeman JE, Johnson S, *et al*. Overview: deinstitutionalisation of psychiatric patients, a critical review of outcome studies. *Am J Psychiatry* 1981;**138**:736-74.
2 Kiesler C. Mental hospitals and alternative care. *Am Psychol* 1982;**4**:354-60.
3 Tessler R, Goldman H. *The chronic mentally ill: assessing the community support program.* Cambridge, Massachusetts: Ballinger, 1982.
4 Anthony W, Cohen M, Farkas M, Cohen B. The chronically mentally ill and case management—more than a response to a dysfunctional system. *Community Ment Health J* 1988;**24**:219-28.
5 Thornicroft G. The concept of case management for long-term mental illness. *Int Rev Psychiatry* 1991;**3**:125-32.
6 Torrey F. Continuous treatment teams in the care of the chronic mentally ill. *Hospital Community Psychiatry* 1986;**37**:1243-7.
7 Patmore C, Weaver T. *Community mental health teams. Lessons for planners and managers.* London: Good Practices in Mental Health, 1991.
8 Renshaw J, Hampson R, Thomason C, Darton R, Judge K, Knapp M. *Care in the community: the first steps.* Aldershot: Gower, 1988.
9 Intagliata J. Improving the quality of care for the chronic mentally disabled: the role of case management. *Schizophrenia Bulletin* 1982;**8**:655-74.
10 Challis D. *Case management in community care.* Aldershot: Gower, 1986.
11 House of Commons. Social Services Committee. *Second report. Session 1984-85. Community care.* London: HMSO, 1985:paragraph 181.
12 Griffiths R. *Community care: an agenda for action.* London: HMSO, 1988:v.
13 Secretaries of State for Health, Social Security, Wales, and Scotland. *Caring for people. Community care in the next decade and beyond.* London: HMSO, 1989:21. (Cm 849.)
14 House of Commons. *The National Health Service and community care act.* London: HMSO, 1990.
15 Department of Health. *The care programme approach for people with a mental illness referred to as the specialist psychiatric services 1990.* London: Department of Health, 1990. (HC(90)23/LASSL(90)11.)
16 Onyett S. *Case management in mental health.* London: Chapman and Hall, 1992.
17 Department of Health, Social Services Inspectorate. *Care management and assessment. Summary of practice guidance.* London: HMSO, 1991.
18 Laming H. *Implementing caring for people. Assessment.* London: Department of Health, 1992.
19 British Medical Association. *Priorities for community care.* London: BMA, 1992.
20 Blom-Cooper L, Murphy E. Mental health services and resources. *Psychiatric Bulletin* 1991;**15**:665-8.

Community psychiatry in Scotland

IAN PULLEN

Background

The implementation of the community care changes throughout the United Kingdom marks the culmination of a series of major health and social care reforms. The avowed aims of achieving value for money and improved consumer choice through the introduction of competitive internal markets have yet to be tested. The political complexion of Scotland means that any proposed change to the NHS has tended to be greeted with a mixture of suspicion and resistance. As a result very few self governing trusts and fundholding general practices exist north of the border. And although Scotland has not had a wide reaching policy of moving psychiatric patients out of hospitals, community care for mentally ill people has advanced spontaneously.

Last October Lord Fraser of Carmyllie, minister of state for health and social work at the Scottish Office, announced what was described as "the last of the major building blocks for full implementation of the government's community care policy"[1] — the finance for provision of community care by local authorities in the coming year. A total of £41m will be transferred from central government to Scottish local authorities in 1993-4 with a further £20m towards implementing assessment and care management. The Mental Illness Specific Grant, which had a tiny budget before 1991, will be increased to £21m.

From the psychiatrist's perspective it is important to remember that these sums are "in support of not only the elderly, mentally ill, mentally handicapped and physically disabled people but also drug and alcohol abusers, homeless persons . . . mothers and babies in registered specialised accommodation, terminally ill people in nursing homes, people on probation and ex-offenders in registered accommodation."[1] The sums of money are large, but so too is the level of need in Scotland.

Scotland has a population of approximately 5 million, most of whom live in or close to cities or towns. An important minority of the population lives in far flung, sparsely populated areas such as the highlands and islands. The provision of psychiatric care to these areas must, necessarily, be different from that for densely populated cities. In rural areas community psychiatric nurses are more autonomous than their urban counterparts and all psychiatric staff have to travel to see patients. This diversity of service presents particular challenges for planning.

Most people with mental illness are treated in the community by general practitioners. But in Scotland, as elsewhere, most of the mental health budget has been consumed by services based at mental hospitals. In recent years psychiatrists in Scotland have peered over the border, somewhat bemused by the speed at which psychiatric long stay beds have been emptied in England. Visiting speakers from England have chided their Scottish colleagues for their slow pace of change, citing bed numbers in Scotland and the building of an entirely new psychiatric hospital in Aberdeen as examples of outmoded practice. In fact such simplistic comparisons are misleading.

Caution is needed when attempting to interpret cross national data on psychiatric hospitals because of many confounding factors, demographic and geographical, as well as the pattern and availability of alternative services. Over the past two decades the resident population in Scottish mental hospitals fell by 20%,[2] but the proportion of residents aged 65 or over rose from 45% in 1970 to 66% by 1988.[3] The number of old and very old people in Scottish psychiatric hospitals accounts for much of the difference in bed numbers on the two sides of the border and reflects the poor provision of local authority run places for elderly confused people in Scotland. For example, in 1985 only 238 places in local authority and registered nursing homes for mentally ill people were recorded in national statistics in Scotland, a shortfall of 1000 places from the number recommended by the government's guidelines.[4]

History of Scottish community care

Despite such criticisms, Scottish mental health services have often been in the vanguard of community care developments, with services evolving locally for pragmatic reasons. But many of these services have not been evaluated effectively. At Dingleton Hospital in the borders a community model based on teams for home visiting and treatment has been used for the scattered population of 100 000 since the 1960s, when Dr Maxwell Jones extended from the hospital his ideas about therapeutic communities.[5,6] Dingleton's practice of seeing all patients in their own homes (or occasionally the general practitioner's surgery) has never been systematically evaluated. Yet this continuing service predates the better known crisis team at Napsbury Hospital, St Albans, by at least eight years.

Scotland has also led the way in moving psychiatrists into primary care. Exactly 40 years ago the first general practice health centre in Scotland was opened at Sighthill in Edinburgh. Three years later the first psychiatric clinics were held at Sighthill.[7] By 1987 more than half of Scottish consultant psychiatrists were spending some time each week in primary care settings[8] compared with fewer than a fifth in England and Wales.[9] This move of resources into the community was entirely unplanned and arose from local initiatives.[8] Because it did not reflect Scottish Office policy its development went unrecorded, such work being undifferentiated from normal outpatient sessions for statistical purposes. This type of work represents a hidden shift of resources into the community[10] because its considerable costs are generally attributed to the budget for psychiatric hospitals.

The development of psychiatric services in Scotland has been influenced greatly by the sites chosen for the Victorian asylums. Many were built on the edge of towns or cities and have subsequently been overtaken by urban development. For example, the Royal Edinburgh Hospital is just 3 km from the city centre in a pleasant residential area (Morningside), and Gartnavel Royal Hospital is on the edge of Glasgow's equivalent suburb (Kelvinside). In England and Wales the policy encompassed in *Hospital Services for the Mentally Ill*[11] sought to overcome the problem caused by the many mental hospitals built at a considerable distance from their catchment populations by opening psychiatric units on district general hospital sites. This policy was not adopted in Scotland, where there are few such psychiatric units. Indeed, a report by a working group of the National Medical Consultative Committee in 1989[12] saw "merit in the development in

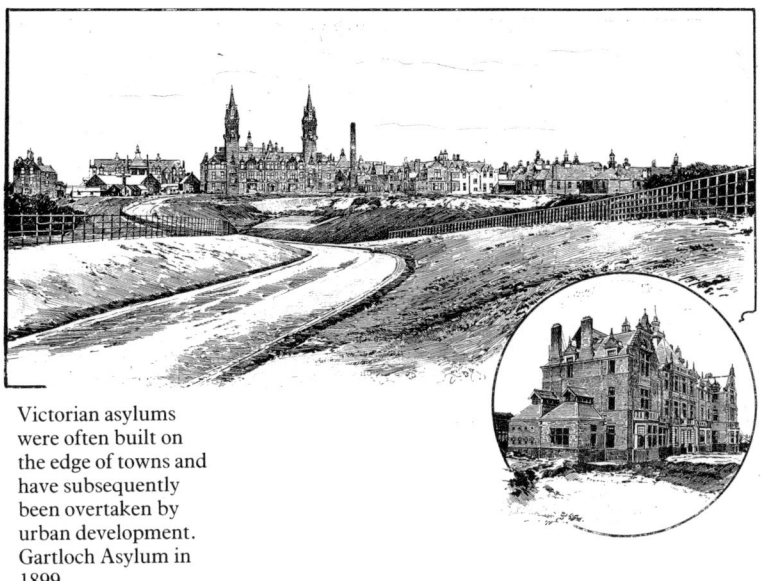

Victorian asylums were often built on the edge of towns and have subsequently been overtaken by urban development. Gartloch Asylum in 1899

Scotland of the concept of inpatient care based on a 'mental health campus'" which would include units for assessment and short term care, medium to long term care, and special facilities for adults with behavioural problems due to brain damage combined with multiple physical disabilities.

In 1980, *Scottish Health Authorities' Priorities for the Eighties* (SHAPE)[4] was published. Care of mentally ill, mentally handicapped, elderly, and elderly mentally disabled people was grouped by the report under category A, which was given priority for health boards' spending. A main objective was to work towards a community based service for people with mental illness through joint planning by the NHS, local authorities, and voluntary agencies. Five years later *Mental Health in Focus* described the mental health services in Scotland as "a deprived area of care" and noted "a serious shortfall, in Scotland, of community alternatives to inpatient mental health care."[13] The report warned that failure to develop comprehensive locally based mental health services "can be remedied only if the necessary initial resources are forthcoming."[13] In 1987 an unpublished report, known as SHARPEN (*Scottish Health Authorities Review of Priorities for the Eighties and Nineties*), pointed out the deficiency of local authority provision for mentally ill people and noted local authorities' particular responsibilities under the Mental Health (Scotland) Act 1984. This report suggested the development of community teams with community psychiatric nurses based in primary care, and health boards were finally persuaded of the desirability of psychiatric units in district general hospitals.

Current problems

Some current problems reflect decisions made many years ago. In the 1970s, when comprehensive resettlement services were first developed and psychiatric wards were emptied by the steady resettlement of low dependency patients into group homes, the opportunity to close beds was not always taken. Instead a growing number of elderly demented people were admitted because of the local authorities' failure to provide alternative care. Thus, low dependency psychiatric patients were replaced by patients who required much higher levels of staffing without a commensurate increase in funding.

Over the past five years the pace of discharges from psychiatric hospitals has accelerated as elderly patients have been transferred to the community. In fact they have been moved into nursing homes funded by the Department of Social Security. This raises the question of what constitutes the community. Do the private "nursing homes" such as that with up to 240 beds on one site proposed for the west of Scotland really count as community care? If such a home places its residents under the care of a consultant psychiatrist, surely it should be called a hospital. If the consultant withdraws and the residents come under the care of a general practitioner, who might from time to time call in a psychiatrist, the home is called a nursing home in the community. This seems similar to the semantic juggling reported by Jones and Poletti when visiting Italy after the introduction of Law 180 in 1978, which forbade the admission of any new patients to mental hospitals.[14] They saw some "family homes" which looked like ordinary mental hospital wards, and although patients in some wards were referred to as "guests," this did not prevent them from being confined by locked doors.

Some former long stay patients have been discharged to supported accommodation run by housing associations and others to hostels. It makes good sense for housing associations to buy several houses in adjoining streets for ease of monitoring and staff support. But these cluster developments have proved unpopular with local residents and with local general practitioners, who often feel relatively unsupported in taking responsibility for up to 20 recently discharged chronically mentally ill people. It is quite clear that community care developments in Scotland have failed to keep pace with discharge of patients and the closure of long stay beds, although the range of facilities has improved together with the liaison between the statutory and voluntary sectors. The number of community psychiatric nurses has increased, but nowhere in Scotland do their numbers approach those in many English districts. Day hospital places have also continued to increase, but in many districts clinical psychology services are underresourced. Finally, the impact of the SHAPE and SHARPEN reports on health boards' spending has been disappointing.

The new reforms

By 1 April 1992 all local authorities and health boards in Scotland were required to produce community care plans. This has led to a closer working relationship, with the adoption of coterminous boundaries between health and social work departments in many areas. Some professional groups, especially general practitioners, felt

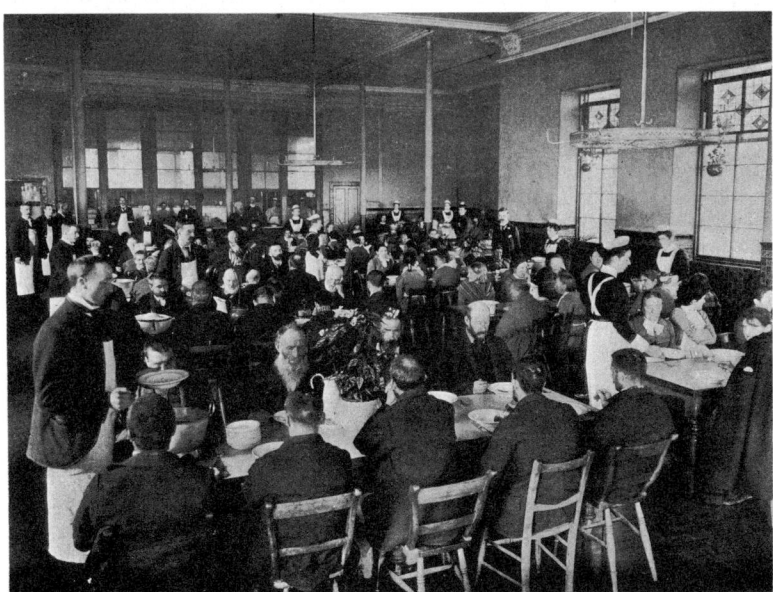

Comprehensive resettlement policies were developed in the 1970s—too late for these patients at Larbert Asylum

that they had been left out of this planning process. To redress the balance the Scottish Office held a workshop in Crieff in June 1992 on the role of the general practitioner in the primary care team. The chief executive of the NHS in Scotland, the chairman of the Scottish General Medical Services Committee (BMA), and 100 general practitioners held a vigorous debate on the need to clarify the role of the general practitioner in the assessment process, the need for training and education, and involvement in the planning process.

In many ways Scotland is in a strong position to benefit from the community care reforms. Because of the slower pace in the rundown of hospital beds than in England, there is a smaller pool of homeless former patients in the community and a larger reservoir of resources in mental hospitals, and now there is a greater possibility of discharging elderly patients to nursing homes. The close working relationship that has developed between psychiatrists and general practitioners[8] should support general practitioners in their role as primary carers for former inpatients. The leave of absence arrangements allowed under section 18 of the Mental Health (Scotland) Act 1984 enable the psychiatrist and mental health officer to ensure a higher level of supervision of vulnerable patients in the community than is permitted under the Mental Health Act 1983. The community supervision orders proposed for England and Wales would permit a similar level of supervision if enacted.[15]

Implications for training

General practitioners already deal with up to 95% of identified psychiatric morbidity in the community without reference to specialist psychiatric services.[16] Increasingly they will be asked to take care of people with more serious mental illnesses. Although vocational training for general practice has been mandatory for almost two decades only 40% of general practitioners registering with the General Medical Council have had a psychiatric attachment. General practitioners will require a higher level of knowledge and expertise in psychiatry than has previously been the case.

Psychiatrists may increasingly be working alongside general practitioners, but there are few training posts in community psychiatry. Consultant psychiatrists in Scotland do, at least, take an equal number of psychiatry trainees when they work in primary care settings.[8] In England and Wales only half of all psychiatrists working in primary care are accompanied by trainees.[9]

Conclusion

Scottish psychiatric services have developed at a different pace and in a somewhat different form from those south of the border. In many ways Scotland is in a strong position to face the challenge posed by the community care reforms. In recent years, however, for financial reasons social work departments have restricted their work almost exclusively to statutory tasks, people with mental health problems having a very low priority. The new lead role for social workers as assessors and purchasers of community care will effectively remove any prospect of direct social work casework with the mentally ill.

The changes, however, come hard on the heels of the introduction of clinical directorates and new unit structures, the NHS internal market, and a reorganisation of social work departments. These reforms, untested by pilot evaluations, represent a leap of faith. It remains to be seen whether they turn out like "hunting the gowk."

A gowk in Scotland is a cuckoo, a Scots equivalent of "un poisson d'avril" in France or an April Fool. Hunting the gowk is a fool's errand.

1 Scottish Office Social Work Services Group. *Community care: resources for 1993-94.* Edinburgh: Scottish Health Services, 1992.
2 Scottish Office. *Scotland's health—a policy statement.* Edinburgh: HMSO, 1992.
3 Information and Statistics Division, Common Services Agency. *Inpatient data 1987 and 1988. (mental illness hospitals, psychiatric units and mental handicap hospitals).* Edinburgh: Scottish Health Services, 1990.
4 Scottish Health Authorities. *Priorities for the eighties.* Edinburgh: HMSO, 1980.
5 Jones D. Community psychiatry in the borders. In: Drucker N, ed. *Creating community mental health services in Scotland.* Vol 2. Edinburgh: Scottish Association for Mental Health, 1987.
6 Jones M. *The process of change. From a closed to an open system in a mental hospital.* London: Routledge and Kegan Paul, 1982.
7 Dean RM. Sighthill—the evolution of a health centre. *J R Coll Gen Pract* 1972; 22:161-8.
8 Pullen IM, Yellowlees AJ. Scottish psychiatrists in primary health care settings: a silent majority. *Br J Psychiatry* 1988;153:663-6.
9 Strathdee G, Williams P. A survey of psychiatrists in primary care: the silent growth of a new service. *J R Coll Gen Pract* 1984;34:615-8.
10 Morgan DH. Hidden spending on community services. *Br J Psychiatry* (in press).
11 *Better services for the mentally ill.* London: HMSO, 1975. (Cmnd 6233.)
12 Working group of National Medical Consultative Committee. *Mental hospitals in focus.* Edinburgh: HMSO, 1989.
13 Scottish Home and Health Department, Scottish Education Department. *Mental health in focus.* Edinburgh: HMSO, 1985.
14 Jones K, Poletti A. Understanding the Italian experience. *Br J Psychiatry* 1985;146:341-7.
15 Public Policy Committee Working Group. *Community supervision orders. A report.* London: Royal College of Psychiatrists, 1993. (Chairman R Bluglass.)
16 Goldberg D, Huxley P. *Mental illness in the community: the pathway to psychiatric care.* London: Tavistock, 1980.
17 Royal College of General Practitioners. *General practitioner vocational training in psychiatry.* London: RCGP, 1993.

Helping disabled people — the user's view

PETER SWAIN

Background

The main needs for most people with physical disabilities are housing and help with daily living. Thus, many of them will find the new emphasis on social aspects of community care particularly relevant. Peter Swain is a disabled man who leads a project in east Devon which ensures that disabled people have a voice in helping to shape the services they need. In this chapter he explains how the project, Living Options East Devon, works and how the new legislation for community care might affect disabled people.

All disabled people would get a good deal if unlimited funding were available for community care. They would have individual assessments of need to identify care packages and equipment required for independent living. Care managers would have the satisfaction of working in a system that allowed them to solve problems and use the skills they had learnt during training. Until recently, the strong Swedish and Danish social welfare systems offered such services with few cost constraints.[1]

But our new world of community care is cash limited. Clearly, priorities will have to be set and only the most pressing needs will be met. People with physical disabilities have certain key priorities for care (see box), the most basic of which is somewhere to live.

Special housing

Without suitable housing, community care for disabled people is doomed to failure. But the government's initial publications on the reforms did not mention housing. Subsequent documents highlighted the need for and lack of adequate "special needs" provision. New building programmes for disabled people have been reduced substantially[2] and the availability of suitable rented accommodation was decimated in the 1980s by the policy that gave council tenants the right to buy their homes.

The lack of housing is lamentable, given the growing numbers of people who have long life expectancy but severe disability after surviving accidents. There are also many more young people who now hope to live independently in the community, rather than in institutions or their parents' homes, after passing through special education. Expectations are growing constantly and packages of care must begin to match them.

Care packages

There is nothing new about care packages. They have been used for years by a few disabled people, but often at huge cost.[3] The concept of care management is not new, either. A similar job has been done for years by good home care organisers who know their patches and can mobilise swiftly a range of services to meet a variety of needs. The reforms simply identify and formalise this role.

Clearly identified care managers could make the process of referral relatively straightforward, predictable, and quick. Effective referral should take into account clients' views on services, and this will depend on good, up to date information on what is available so that clients can make informed choices. Social services departments must

---

Priorities for disabled people
- Somewhere to live
- Appropriate care services
- Mobility
- Access
- Opportunity

ensure that such information is readily available. They must also decide on realistic minimum standards and time intervals for responding to referrals, setting up assessments, and initiating packages of care.

Assessment should be a joint exercise, with disabled people and,

---

Case study 1

Mrs A is a young woman with multiple sclerosis living with her teenage daughter in an adapted council bungalow. She uses a wheelchair. Her care package is provided by a private agency, social services, and health services.

Mrs A receives money from the Independent Living Fund, all of which she pays to the private agency that provides the bulk of her care. She has to supplement this cost from other sources, and also receives some help from the Multiple Sclerosis Society.

The private agency staff sleep in with Mrs A five nights a week, and social services provide a home care assistant for two nights. The agency provides a carer for two hours each morning and for two hours in the afternoon at weekends. Social services provide a home care assistant for two hours every weekday afternoon. The district nurse calls once a morning on weekdays to help Mrs A to the toilet. "Perhaps they think I go into suspended animation for the rest of the time!"

Mrs A speaks very highly of the private agency, saying that it has never let her down and that she can even telephone in the middle of the night if she needs help. She feels the agency has taken particular trouble to match her carers to her individual needs and preferences, and is happy with the small team of staff who work for her.

She speaks less highly of the social services department, saying that she would prefer to be given the money equivalent of their input so that she could purchase all her care from one source. Social services does not seem to have the flexibility to match client and carer satisfactorily, and she is concerned that she has to adjust to different carers from week to week.

Mrs A regards the proprietor of the private agency as her care manager, although a part time social worker, one of the local home care managers, and the general practitioner are very much involved in her case. Case conferences are held at irregular intervals.

Sorting out a care package is "a free for all, you take the best you can," says Mrs A. "It really is a do it yourself job, and it is very difficult. I really had to be determined to get this package together. I can't remember who told me about the Independent Living Fund, perhaps it was the private agency. That was all processed fairly quickly. On the whole, I feel that social services and health will only do what they have to do, and no more."

when appropriate, their carers participating. They will be in the best position to ensure that their other essential needs—access, mobility, and opportunity—are provided for along with housing and domiciliary support. These "value added" factors open the way to further and higher education, employment, personal relationships, and all those other things that contribute to an acceptable quality of life. Ignoring these factors during assessment would reduce considerably the potential benefits of the new system and would leave many disabled people unfulfilled and unnecessarily limited.

Thus, good holistic care management could help the overall development of disabled people's potential. Some people might want to act as their own care managers, although they would probably need training to acquire the skills needed to employ and organise teams of care staff.

As well as providing for clients' basic needs and potentials, care packages must be responsive, flexible, and reliable (see case study 1). Whenever possible a single agency should provide the bulk of care. This approach is less intrusive for clients, cheaper to provide, and less bureaucratic to administer than a multiagency package.[4] When many services are provided, they must be coordinated properly—having staff stacking up at the door waiting to do the next job is almost as frustrating as having no one turn up.

Finally, what about the frustrations of the care managers? Who should care for them? Their jobs will often be stressful and they might benefit from a neutral forum in which to discuss their concerns and tensions.

Monitoring care

The new policy for community care assumes that huge numbers of agencies and individuals are ready to provide services. But this assumption may not yet be true in all parts of Britain. The number and range of services should be expanding because social services departments are now obliged to buy in 85% of services from the independent sector. The growth of the private sector will inevitably follow the supply of cash. Will purchasers be able to monitor and sustain the quality of private care?

Disabled users will be looking for safeguards against poor services and against packages that are driven by cost alone (see case study 2). Private and, for that matter, voluntary agencies offering care should be subject to regular and rigorous quality checks. They will have to set

HELPING DISABLED PEOPLE—THE USER'S VIEW

> ### Case study 2
> G is a young man who has had multiple sclerosis for most of his adult life. After his mother died he went into residential care. After about two years he moved out into an adapted local authority bungalow with a complex care network to sustain him—this involved support from the voluntary organisation Crossroads, community nurses, home helps, and private agencies. He spent regular periods in local respite facilities for treatment and maintenance care.
>
> In time the package became too difficult to maintain because of the intensity of care needed and because of G's deteriorating psychological condition. Extra care was bought from a private agency using money from the Independent Living Fund, supplemented by direct cash payments from the local home help budget.
>
> The agency contracted to provide the care was new and was one of the cheapest locally, offering the highest number of care hours for the money available. One of its conditions of service was that no other agency could provide support.
>
> All of G's affairs were conducted on his behalf by staff from the agency. They arranged his respite care and holidays, booking transport as necessary. But it soon became apparent that the transport was being arranged to suit the agency, with early morning departures and late evening returns. The transport service became suspicious of the agency's motives and eventually withdrew its vehicles. Further concerns arose when the agency asked social services to pay for a leather restraining harness for G so that he could be left alone safely, saving on care hours and costs.
>
> At this point the voluntary organisation Living Options was called in by G's social worker. A case conference was held and the agency's input is being carefully monitored.

themselves minimum standards and expect scrutiny by independent inspectors. Users' groups should also help in auditing quality and customer satisfaction.

Complaints procedures are often inadequate. People are often loath to complain because they do not want to be ungrateful or do not have any faith in the likely redress for poor service. At the very least users should be able to expect that providers who fail quality assurance checks will not be contracted with again.

The voluntary sector, that amorphous and uncoordinated mass of services and pressure groups, will also have to be monitored. And it will need to prepare itself to play a big part in what the community care gurus call "the mixed economy of care," acquiring skills in management, administration, and contracting to convince potential purchasers that the "goods" will be delivered on time.

The new arrangements will have a profound effect on the voluntary sector. A few voluntary organisations are very large and professional and are managed as well as, if not better than, their counterparts in the statutory health and social services. Most, however, are small and not well run. Those organisations that cannot respond to the new system's demands in imaginative and flexible ways may not survive. Those that can rise to the challenge will be a great asset to the provider network. But purchasers must resist the temptation to tamper with them and jeopardise the independence that makes them special.

Fitting together purchasers and providers from the various sectors can be very complicated. In east Devon a special coordinating agency, Living Options, acts as a link between agencies, sorts out the planning and delivery of care, and ensures that service users are right at the centre of the planning process.

Living Options—east Devon

East Devon is a relatively rural district stretching from Okehampton in the west to Axminster in the east, some 60 miles away. The district has quite a small population of about 300 000, mainly concentrated in Exeter, yet it has more than 150 voluntary groups for people with disabilities. Trying to pull these groups together to form a coherent consumer voice is a daunting task. Many of them want to concentrate on their own sectional interests and many think parochially, looking to Exeter for guidance only reluctantly.

When we tried to establish Living Options as an informal confederation to represent disabled people the sceptics poured cold water on our plans. All too often, they said, voluntary organisations raise their heads over the parapet only to carp and criticise. Living Options set out to work in the boardroom, not at the barricades.

We have a clear vision of our aims and methods. And we fell into a fertile climate in which Exeter health authority had closed its institutions for mental illness and learning disability and had initiated high quality community services to replace them. Focusing on physically disabled people next was a logical step.

The Living Options project was launched in January 1990, funded mainly by the Nuffield Provincial Hospitals Trust. We were also helped greatly by an annual grant from the health authority, which

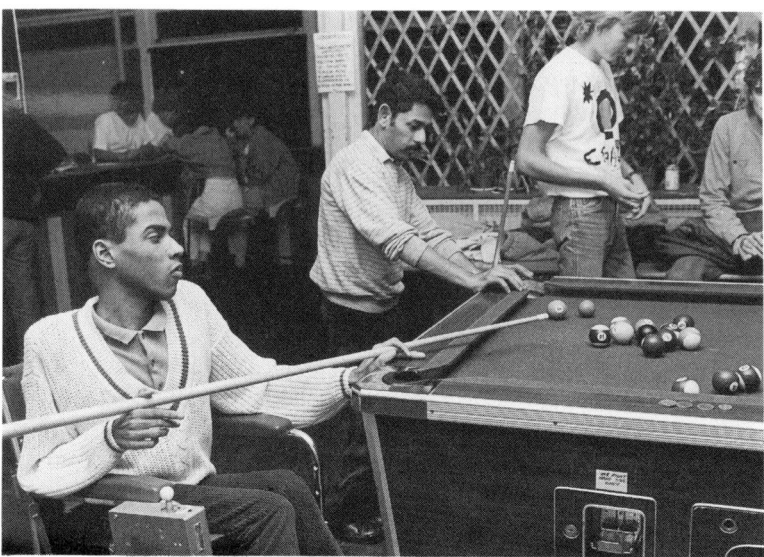

Mobility, access, and opportunity are essential to develop an acceptable quality of life

paid for the hire of a suitable meeting room at a local hotel, travel expenses, and publication costs for reports.

Several years of planning and work before we started up had already produced a county wide federation of services that provide information on disability. In 1990 Living Options began a general survey of what services actually do. We also set up a subgroup of users and carers to work with the Disablement Services Centre in Exeter and help assimilate wheelchair services into the NHS.[5] The local managers took up many of our recommendations and continue to collaborate with us about wheelchair services. And another district, seeing that we had solved a difficult problem, adopted our plan verbatim.

The subgroup went on to commission a three month trial of lightweight wheelchairs,[6] which expanded the range issued by the disablement services centre and increased purchasers' flexibility. Now we are trying to develop the centre's range of equipment even further by espousing the voucher scheme recommended in the McColl report[7] and to open a showroom where disabled people can be assessed for non-standard equipment. These early successes showed that Living Options could help users to participate in decision making as equal partners.

Subsequent work has focused on problems shown up by our first survey of services. Last year we pulled together the findings in a report, *Pathways to Quality Services*,[4] which is now being used by health and social services as a basis for planning and purchasing.

We have also undertaken more specialised work. In August 1991 we published a report on the needs of 100 people (16-65 years) with arthritis,[8] which was taken up quickly by local planners. Another special report on people with sensory impairment will be published soon, and we have already linked with the district's audiology strategy group and among other things identified a shortfall in lip reading classes.

As well as drawing together information, Living Options is affecting local policy in two other ways—by acting as a watchdog and by taking part in planning at a high level. Firstly, we discovered a worrying lack of registration or monitoring of private care agencies, which could leave disabled people open to abuse. With two reputable private care employers and representatives from many interested agencies we drafted a voluntary code of practice which purchasers could use to accredit private providers. And some of our members have now joined the social services inspectorate to put together clear guidelines on accreditation. Finally, we are starting regular audit of randomly picked cases to monitor customer satisfaction with community care policies.

When Living Options started up, various attempts had been made to revamp services for physical disability in east Devon, without any real impact. Some new initiatives had been set up through individual effort with haphazard funding: inevitably they failed when initial finances were withdrawn or frozen. Exeter still lacked a cohesive plan for disability, and managers in health and social services had little idea of what might be included. To resolve this a joint disability forum of senior managers from health, social services, and housing was set up. Living Options was invited to elect three representatives to sit on the forum and in 1991 the chairman of the Living Options Working Party was appointed chairman of the forum. Consumers were now clearly taking a leading role.

Conclusions

The main effect of the Living Options project in east Devon has been effective collaboration between statutory and voluntary agencies. The community care reforms will mean that agencies throughout Britain will have to collaborate in similar ways. While the mechanisms of joint planning will be familiar to many, joint working—passing referrals, swapping caseloads, and establishing networks of expertise—will be almost universally new.

If new services are to be sensitive to users' needs then disabled people must be included at the earliest stages of consultation and planning. The reforms will not mean much if they do not lead to tangibly improved care. Most users will not be concerned with the finer points of needs assessment, care plans, and care packages, but if the hands on service is no better than before they will want to know why.

1 Swain P. *A Scandinavian study tour of services for physically disabled people.* Exeter: Exeter Council for Independent Living, 1988.
2 Housing Corporation. *Housing for people with disabilities: the needs of wheelchair users.* London: Housing Corporation, 1991.
3 Fielder B. *Living options lottery: housing and support services for people with severe disabilities, 1986-88.* London: Prince of Wales Advisory Group, 1988.
4 Howe M, Swain P. *Pathways to quality services. A review of residential, housing, support and day services in the Exeter health district.* Exeter: Living Options, 1992.
5 Living Options Working Party. *Wheelchair services operational policy.* Exeter: Living Options, 1990.
6 Living Options Working Party. *Lightweight wheelchair trial: a user's view.* Exeter: Living Options, 1991.
7 McColl I. *Review of artiicial limb and appliance centre services.* London: Department of Health and Social Security, 1986.
8 Murray T, Howe M. *A survey of services for younger people with arthritis in the Exeter health district.* Exeter: Living Options, 1991.

Mental health services — the user's view

PETER CAMPBELL

Background

The needs of people with serious mental illnesses have dominated much of the debate on reforming community care. In this article Peter Campbell, who has used mental health services many times in the past, explains how the reforms could affect people like him. He welcomes the thinking behind the changes, particularly the idea that people who use community care should take part in planning services, but he warns that implementing the new philosophy might prove very difficult. Mr Campbell is secretary of a voluntary organisation for users of mental health services called Survivors Speak Out. The views he expresses here are his own, and do not necessarily reflect those of Survivors Speak Out.

The past three months have proved difficult times for community mental health care policy. As the starting date for the final and most substantial series of reforms approaches there are still major doubts and fears about the practicality and desirability of the changes. The much publicised case of Ben Silcock[1] and the health secretary's response to it[2] have once again revealed important differences among mental health care providers about which care is most necessary; it has also emphasised underlying uncertainties about whether community care for people with a diagnosis of severe mental illness can ever really work. A favourable consensus may still exist, but it carries a rather battered look.

In the face of such doubts a large number of mental health service users, including me, remain resolutely in favour of community care. We believe it is not only a viable option but the only option that can lead to significant changes in our status, as recipients of services and as citizens. We know that community care is no panacea and we share current anxieties that, without proper resources, institutionalisation may be replaced by neglect. But it is hard to see how the wider transformations we seek can be established except on the foundations that community mental health services could provide. In these circumstances our concerns are not that community care changes are a step too far, but that they will not go far enough to produce radical change.

Changing the location of care

It is certainly true that the location of care is changing. Community mental health care does imply the closure of the large, asylum style psychiatric hospitals, not least because many of the resources for new services are tied up in the old institutions. Closures have been taking place over the past 10 years. Soon the speed and scope of the closure programme will increase. A recent survey by the National Schizophrenia Fellowship has shown that 45 psychiatric hospitals will close by the year 2000.[3]

Hospital closures are major events in the lives of many users. As someone who has been admitted into psychiatric care 16 times in the past 25 years and has usually received acute care in asylum style settings, I shed few tears for the disappearance of these places. While I do not dismiss the care and treatment I have received during those admissions, I did not have to spend many weeks in the "old bins" to become aware of their shortcomings as therapeutic environments. The isolation—I have only once been in an admission ward less than a dozen miles from my home—and the physical environment— inappropriate design, upstairs dormitories that must be locked all day, uninvolving regimentation—are aspects of a system of care whose inadequacies should not be underestimated.

Moreover, while there are good reasons for concern about the availability of services for "revolving door patients" during the run down of the old psychiatric hospitals and while doubts remain over the capacity of district general hospital units to provide appropriate care to people in crisis, the relocation of the long stay population of psychiatric hospitals is achieving some successful results. There is evidence to support the anecdotal impression that long stay patients

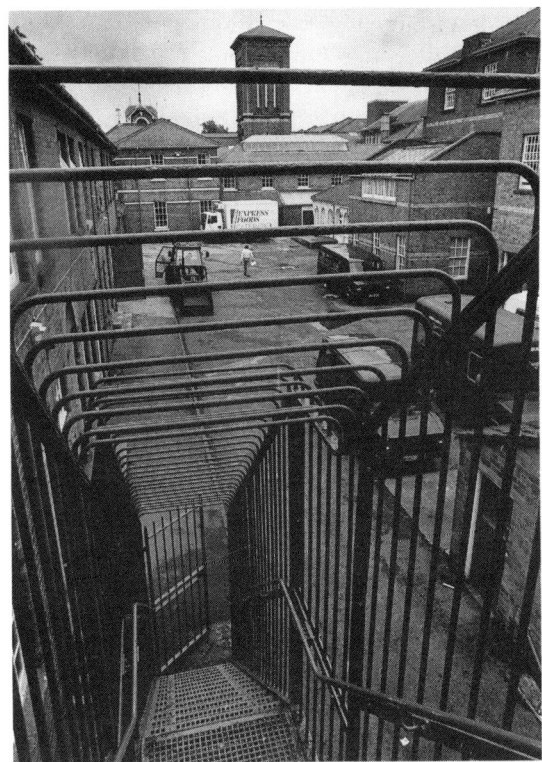

You don't have to spend long in an old psychiatric hospital to be aware of the environment's shortcomings

both prefer and are capable of living in community settings. Monitoring of people moved from Friern Hospital in north London and Claybury Hospital in Essex shows that they are not slipping out of the system and are enjoying a better quality of life with greater independence and a more varied social life.[4] With adequate resourcing and well designed support systems, relocation can enhance lives.

But the community care reforms imply more than a shift in the location of care. According to the government's rhetoric, a fundamental change in the relationship between the provider and the recipient of care and treatment will transform the nature of services themselves. Thus the 1990 NHS and Community Care Act promises us a new approach to service provision that puts the needs of users and carers first. At the very least individuals will become consumers rather than recipients of care. At best their rights as equal citizens will be acknowledged and secured. While service providers are struggling to address "needs led assessment," "individualised care packages," and "care management" service users are beguiled with talk of "increased choice," "user involvement," and "patient empowerment." It is clear that something important is supposed to be happening. But what does it really mean? Behind the rhetoric, is the power of users, either as individuals or as an interest group, actually increasing?

Users are important

The role of users within the mental health system has developed rapidly over the past 10 years. Although the relation between the growth of action by organised groups of service users and the increasing importance of health service consumerism is not straightforward, the shift towards community care and the ideological changes accompanying it have undoubtedly given users the opportunity to become important stakeholders. In 1983, at the time of the introduction of the new Mental Health Act, seen then and now as a breakthrough for patients' rights, users were barely involved in the mental health debate. Users were also comparatively powerless within

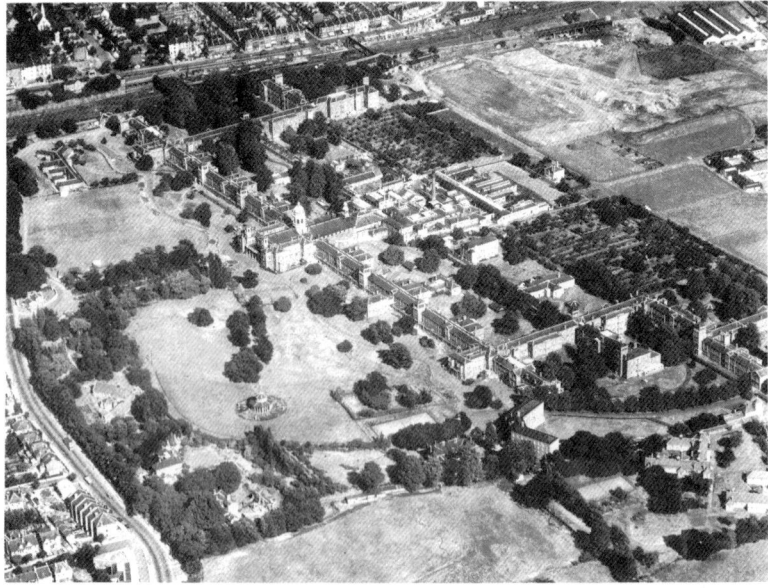

People moved from Friern Hospital in north London are enjoying a better quality of life with greater independence and a more varied social life

mental health voluntary organisations. Independent organisations of users were notable by their absence.

In 1993 there are more than 150 independent organisations of users in the United Kingdom. Major voluntary organisations like MIND and the National Schizophrenia Fellowship work alongside these groups, both locally and nationally, and have adapted their own structures to represent users more effectively. The Community Care Support Force and the Mental Health Task Force—two recently established government initiatives—both have user representation. Up to half a dozen years ago any invitation by the government that offered users meaningful involvement in planning community care would have been seen as unrealistic and even cynical. In current circumstances such involvement is at least a genuine possibility.

Even so there are no grounds for easy optimism. All the evidence available points to the difficulty of involving users effectively in planning processes. Research on the involvement of disabled people in preparing local authorities' community care plans in April 1992 illustrates some of the barriers.[5] Only one in eight local authorities had consulted disabled people before preparing a draft plan. No social services department had produced a plan accessible to people with learning difficulties. There was insufficient recognition that some of the voluntary organisations who helped with the plans do not adequately consult disabled people.

At the same time there are a series of practical problems affecting all consultation with users. Service users are rarely paid for their time. The conduct of meetings often excludes, alienates, or marginalises user representatives. The representativeness of service users' involvement is questioned far beyond that of other interest groups. Although the desire to involve users in planning and consultation is real enough, the unfriendliness of planning structures is not yet sufficiently recognised. Effective involvement in the future may depend not only on more extensive support for user representatives but on overhauling the planning process.

What users can do

It is possible that influencing purchasers of mental health services will prove the most direct way of changing services. In Newcastle a mental health consumer group has been working closely with purchasers over the past two years. The group participates at all stages of the process, including defining needs, revising draft contacts, monitoring existing services through visits or surveys, and contributing to planning future services. The group is already achieving some success, both in altering the detailed specifications in contracts and in challenging longer term mental health strategy. Considerable funding has been found to support the effective functioning of the Newcastle group. Perhaps purchasers or providers elsewhere would not be prepared to devote the necessary resources to involving service users in this way. Experience in Newcastle suggests it could be money well spent.

I believe it is unrealistic to expect the community care reforms to transform services according to the wishes of service users. There may be more room for choice in the new system and users may be in a stronger position to influence the planning of those choices, but the range of services is unlikely to widen. Notable differences remain between what user organisations are demanding and what service providers are willing to provide.

Despite 10 years of pressure for 24 hour, non-medical crisis services such facilities hardly exist in this country. In an era of choice and "needs driven" care, adequate support for people wishing to withdraw from major tranquillisers is not only absent but opposed. Funding restrictions may be partly responsible for these absences, but they also reflect the mental health system's capacity to resist new responses to mental distress. Community care will not circumvent this and will not automatically produce care and treatment that is any less reliant on medication as a therapeutic tool. These are not new issues; nor are they the only important issues for users. But there is a danger that the current reforms will leave untouched fundamental assumptions about the lives and needs of service users.

What will happen to users?

What about the individual users? Will their power increase even if the character of services remains substantially unchanged? Will they have more control over their own care and treatment?

The new arrangements should provide more occasions when mental health workers sit down with individuals to discuss their care in a structured way. The care programme approach introduced in April 1991 for people discharged from hospital and the individual needs assessments to be performed by care managers will permit greater involvement. But it is currently unclear how comprehensive these new procedures will be. A preliminary study by Research and

Development for Psychiatry found that a quarter of health authorities had not implemented the care programme approach. In some districts it has been impossible to make it available to everyone. Care management is being introduced gradually and is focusing on those who are particularly vulnerable or need a wide range of services. Evidence from pilot projects shows the real potential of care management to create flexible care and support controlled by the user.[6]

Advocacy and representation

Real choices are informed choices, and the provision of good independent advocacy and information services will be essential to the effectiveness of the reforms. Advocacy means representing and pursuing someone else's interests as if they were your own. The importance of advocacy in mental health services has been emphasised by the government and this has been reflected in a growth in advocacy projects such as patients' councils and schemes for individual advocates in hospitals. But advocacy services are not welcomed universally. They threaten change in the day to day practice of mental health workers and require a reframing of one to one relationships with clients. As a result it is perhaps not surprising that new advocacy schemes can be viewed with suspicion or seen as "troublemaking." Even where advocacy projects have been established, staff may feel that these are experimental embellishments to services rather than key elements of a new style of care.

In these circumstances the absence of full legal rights to advocacy and representation is particularly unfortunate. The government's refusal fully to implement the Disabled Person's (Services, Consultation and Representation) Act 1986 leaves users dependent on the good practice of service providers, without clear cut rights to assessment or explanation when services are not provided. Without a legal basis for users' role in the assessment process, without full rights to user representation, and without national minimum standards for community care, any increase in users' individual power may be illusory.

There is a danger of overestimating the impact of the community care reforms on the everyday lives of people with a diagnosis of mental illness. As consumers of a health and social care system, our range of choice and our control of our own care may be extended. But these gains will be limited. As citizens in the community, we may find no change at all. In the past few weeks the government has once again blocked an attempt to give disabled people legal protection against discrimination.[7] The destructive poverty ruling the lives of people dependent on benefits is likely to continue and may grow worse. We may be becoming more visible. Will we be less marginal? The community care reforms have been linked with changes in attitudes within mental health services. Their significance to service users will depend on transferring such change to the wider society.

1 Wallace M. Tortured world of the man in the lions' den. *Daily Mail* 1993 Jan 2.
2 Bluglass R. Maintaining the treatment of mentally ill people in the community. *BMJ* 1993;306:159-60.
3 Groves T. Government lacks data on mental hospital closures. *BMJ* 1993;306: 475-6.
4 Thornicroft G, Gooch C, Dayson D. The TAPS project 17: readmissions to hospital for long term psychiatric patients after discharge in the community. *BMJ* 1992;305:996-8.
5 Bewley C, Glendinning G. *Involving disabled people in community care planning.* York: Joseph Rowntree Foundation, 1992. (University of Manchester social care research findings No 27.)
6 Sone K. The luck of the draw. *Community Care* 1992 Jan 30:18-20.
7 Headlines. No civil rights for Britain's disabled people. *BMJ* 1993;306:604.

Old people's homes — the relative's view

MAVIS NICHOLSON, DOROTHY WHITE

Background

On 1 April 1993 new arrangements came into force for arranging and funding residential care for elderly people in Britain. From now on those who seem to need full time care will be assessed first by care managers employed by local authority social services departments. This may lead to admission to an old people's home or a nursing home.

Local authorities have been told to consult both users and carers about such decisions. But what about relatives who have not actually been giving care directly?

The Relatives Association was set up last year as a voluntary organisation for the relatives and friends of older people living in residential homes. Below, its vice president, Mavis Nicholson, a journalist and broadcaster whose mother died of Alzheimer's disease in a residential home last year, gives her personal view of being such a relative. And Dorothy White, the association's founder, explains what the future may hold for elderly residents and their relatives.

A home for mother

Moving someone you love from your home into a Home can never be anything less than upsetting. It is a big decision even when it is a necessary one. For some people it is traumatic, however much they tell themselves it is for the best.

OLD PEOPLE'S HOMES — THE RELATIVES' VIEW

My sister and I were racked with guilt — brain washed, I think, by past notions of old people's homes. They were little better than workhouses, parish run, where unloved nuisances were abandoned. Only heartless children put their parents into them to exist, neglected, until they died. We should surely have got rid of such hang ups by now. But many 60 year olds like myself still have to fight down these very real imaginings.

I sincerely hope my children will not have to fight them when my time comes. I'll leave them a letter of permission, for one thing, taking the onus off them. And, for another, I hope to put my name down for a good home while I'm still capable of making the choice. Ideally I would like to do some voluntary work in the one I have my eye on, so that I'd feel at home there even before I took up residence.

The search for the right home for my mother was gruelling. My sister did most of the groundwork, working on gut reaction, but she found she had little choice. The home we eventually settled on was in fact the only one we could feel positive about. It did not smell of urine, was nicely furnished like a family hotel, and was run by people who seemed naturally affectionate.

But then we came up against some snags in ourselves. My sister was absolutely exhausted from looking after our mother. I felt bad because I hadn't done much of that and here was I about to do even less.

The worst thing about putting your relative in a home is suddenly seeing the person you love in a communal sitting room with all the others who are just like her. On her own, in my sister's house, my mother hadn't seemed pathetic. The privacy had given her some dignity. Now the multiplication struck me as ludicrous, and she was diminished and exposed by it. It had nothing to do with the home itself. I had to make myself get over this reaction. This was life.

Another terrible shock came when I arrived to find my mother wearing something that didn't belong to her. I wasn't alone in this. I remember seeing a staid old gent, whom I'd got to know, appear one afternoon in bright turquoise trousers. And just as I was thinking that with his wits about him he would have died rather than be seen in them, his sister walked in and nearly had forty fits.

As a visitor to an old people's home you already feel bewildered — slightly lost in trying to keep your relationship going with someone who has, in a sense, been taken over by other people. But to see them dressed out of character is too much. Staff can't know exactly how their residents used to dress. So they really should ask relatives to tell them. Labelling clothes and sticking to them is an obvious answer.

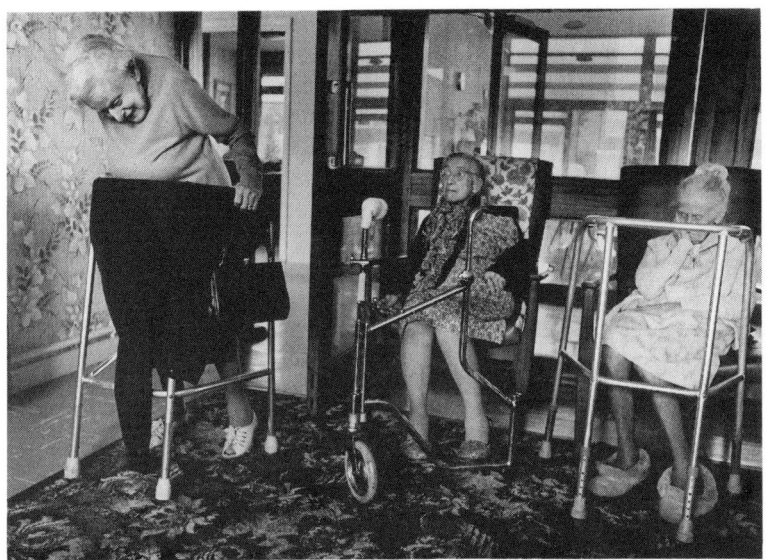

Care in a residential home is often the best solution for a problem with no ideal solutions

One Easter the staff at the home bought everyone a new cardigan for the holiday—a nice gesture. But my mother's was a colour she would never have chosen in a million years and it clashed with all her own clothes.

It is easy to feel you have lost any relative who goes into a residential home, anyway. You can hardly ever do anything for them. Keeping up a conversation is dire. No wonder other members of the family stop visiting them. They feel spare.

And they feel more guilt. You have failed to look after this lost person to the very end, especially in the case of a mother, who had looked after you from the beginning.

Building bridges, making changes

The ordeal is worse for people who, like my sister, have been full time carers. She says she didn't know what hit her when our mother went into the home. She felt isolated. The purpose in her life (even though it had been wearing her out) had gone. Previously her days had been filled with the bath nurse arriving, Meals on Wheels sometimes, the ambulance driver taking mother to the day centre, the day centre staff when she picked up my mother. Then, overnight, everything changed. No visitors arrived. And when she went to the home to see her mother, there was nothing for her to do, although she used to do everything.

There are not anything like enough bridges between those who run homes and those who visit. Similarly, before parent teacher associations were formed, there were no links in schools between teachers and parents. Old people's homes could learn from their lesson.

One of the first things relatives could change is the baby talk in which staff speak to residents. It maybe that staff use this language because they are young and fresh from talking to their own babies like this. Or maybe it's because they are setting up a barrier between themselves and the sorry plight of the people they are caring for day by day.

It is well intended, I'm pretty sure. But I saw it baffling my mother. She looked around to see which infant or puppy they were addressing. She'd answer very primly at first, as if to ward it off.

I worried that it hastened her surrender to being a helpless little thing. But old age is not, in my view, a second childhood. My mother's Alzheimer's disease took away her ability to think who she was, but she was still Olive Irene Mainwaring, an adult who had been a bright and thinking woman in her day.

The Relatives Association

The Relatives Association was set up last year to give the relatives and friends of elderly people in residential care and nursing homes a chance to voice their views on the care given. Many relatives have feelings of isolation, guilt, and frustration which they do not know how to channel. Yet relatives are often able to make sure that care in a residential home is of really good quality and that the individuality of elderly residents is understood and maintained. Many want to do more to help and want to be more aware of the way in which residential homes are run.

Many relatives find that staff are always under pressure, are not well paid, and have very little training. Most relatives are grateful for the concern and kindness shown by the staff. Some worry that they are entrusting their elderly people to a system in which the circumstances of managing homes seem to work against providing the quality and individuality of care they hope for. Yet the fees for residential care often seem enormous and way beyond the limits now covered for residents by income support.

Elderly residents are usually much too frail to be active consumers, but their relatives can take up these issues on their behalf. With this in mind, the Relatives Association was founded. Its main aims are
- to provide an organisation through which relatives can work together with residential homes to maintain and improve the quality of care for older people;
- to provide advice and support to relatives;
- to help develop local groups or networks of relatives;
- to provide a voice for relatives, both locally and nationally.

The first year

During the first year the bulk of the association's work has been to provide an advice and information service. Much of this is done through listening to relatives who telephone for help. It has been possible to help people reconcile themselves to their own feelings of guilt and to talk through their worries about the care of their elderly relatives. Often they find it difficult to take things up with homes. The association helps relatives to sort out what they would like to see changed and gives them the understanding and backing to discuss this with the home's staff.

Most relatives contacting the association do not seem to want to make a formal complaint—although sometimes this may be necessary. They recognise that a home is a living community and that all those concerned—the residents, the staff, the management, and the relatives—have to work together. But more than anything, the relatives want to cease being mere visitors, always on the outside. They want to be brought into the inside.

By responding to consultation documents from the Department of Health, through publications and conferences, and through discussion with owners of residential homes, the association has tried to create a climate of understanding not only of the importance of the continued involvement of their families when older people go into homes, but also of the value of making sure they are able to express their views about the many issues surrounding the provision of care in homes. Relatives may no longer be direct carers (and, indeed, some may never have been carers before the residents went into the homes), but they are usually deeply concerned and are usually the most frequent visitors in homes. They can and do observe what goes on, but they are seldom consulted.

During its first year the association has conducted a pilot study of what relatives thought were the good and not so good features of

OLD PEOPLE'S HOMES—THE RELATIVES' VIEW

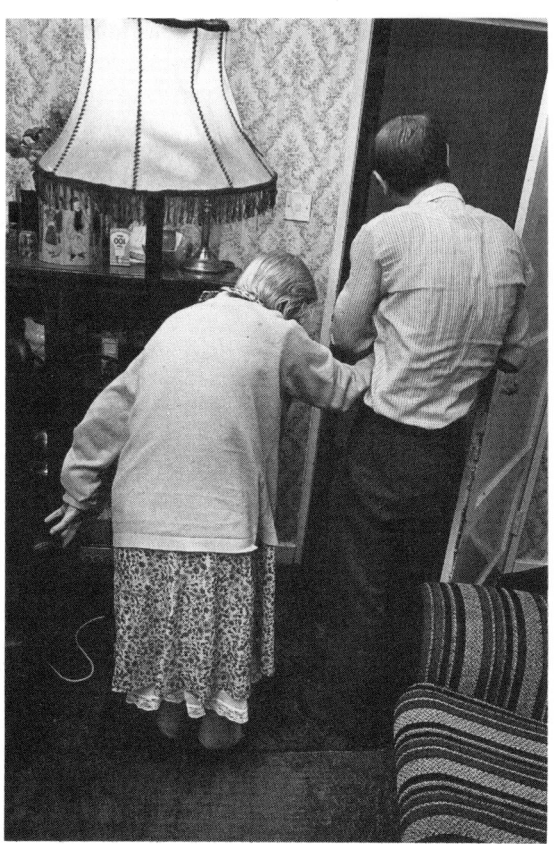

Some elderly people are too frail to be active consumers

residential homes and of their views about residents' reactions to being in homes.[1] We are now working on three booklets which will help relatives to understand better the basic principles and aims in running a home, and which will help both relatives and homes in the difficult task of building up groups of relatives and friends (analogous to schools' parent teacher associations) to work constructively with the home and its staff.

The next task is to help the formation of these groups and of local support networks of relatives. The association does not necessarily intend to start local branches unless this is what local people want; the aim is to get discussion going with local authorities, associations of residential home owners, councils for voluntary service, and local branches of voluntary organisations such as Age Concern, Carers National, and the Alzheimer's Disease Society.

The community care reforms

How does all this fit in with the new arrangements for community care? We hope that the reforms will provide additional flexibility which will help elderly people to remain in their own homes if this is what they want. Our small pilot study of 65 relatives showed that elderly people tend to feel that being in a residential home is at best a necessary decision.[1]

But full time care at home, if that has to imprison a member of the family for several years, may not be a good solution either. Elderly people needing full time care are usually 85 or older and their children are usually in their late 50s and 60s. Half a century ago the ratio of 50-60 year olds to those over 85 was 14:1; now the proportion is 5:1. This is a profound change which puts the pressure of family caring on very few people. This pressure could be increased by a climate of opinion that expects 50-70 year olds to take on the full time care of their aging parents.

Husbands and wives will probably want to go on looking after each other for as long as they possibly can, but the situation may be different for children. The offspring of very elderly people may not be in the best of health, nor may their spouses. They often have other family responsibilities. And some may want some time to lead their own lives before old age overtakes them or to make their contributions to society in different ways from undertaking the full time care of a parent. Finally, there are very real problems when families have never got on well with each other at close quarters. This is why, for many frail elderly residents and their families, care in a home has seemed the best solution for a problem for which there are no ideal solutions.

There are national economic factors that worry relatives, too. Gradually, because income support is given within strict limits, relatives have been pushed into contributing to fees when the residents have used up all their own money. Many relatives can no longer rely on a trickle down of inheritance; they have to contribute from their own resources. It remains to be seen whether this will still happen in the future for residents whose places are purchased by local authorities.

The issue for the future which very much concerns the association is the need to recognise that care in residential homes must still be a part of community care for elderly people who can no longer remain in their own homes. There may be different ways of providing residential care: through smaller units; through arrangements in which relatives and friends do some of the caring; and through closer links with day services so that very old people can attend residential homes regularly before becoming residents. Two major issues are the best way to look after people with Alzheimer's disease and the division between residential care and nursing homes.

The relatives of those in residential homes not only have a great deal to contribute to maintaining present standards of care; many have insights to offer about the future. They should be involved in planning and monitoring, not only for their parents or spouses or friends now, but for their own sakes in the future. One of the tasks of the Relatives Association is to ensure that they are able to make that contribution.

The association was fortunate in starting its life within the auspices of Counsel and Care, a major charity working on behalf of older people. This helped in the initial applications for funding and provided a base. The association now has its own separate charity registration but will maintain links with Counsel and Care. It must, however, pay its way. The association now has a grant from the Department of Health to cover part of its costs and some charitable trust funding, but the greater part of the work of running the association and of developing locally must come through voluntary effort. Retired people who are used to organising things, and who are, or have been, "relatives" are urgently required to assist in this.

Those who are interested in finding out more about the association, or have help to offer, should write to the Relatives Association, Twyman House, 16 Bonny Street, London NW1 9PG, or telephone 071 284 2541.

1 White DM. *Relative views*. London: Relatives Association, 1993.

Index

Page numbers of figures are given in *italics*

advocacy 111–12
Age Concern 27, 37–8
agencies, independent 9
  monitoring 103
  see also contracts
Alcohol Concern 16
alcohol misusers 16, 84
All-Wales Strategy for Mental Handicap 21
All-Wales Strategy for Mental Illness 21
Allen, Molly 41
Alzheimer's disease 116, 120
Armstrong, Graham 61–2
arthritis 103
assessment 7
  Bassetlaw 33-5
  before hospital discharge 10, 34–5, 50–1
  Camberwell 83
  Devon 71
  of disabled people 98–9
  mental health 80–2
  Newcastle 58–61, 63–4
  Northern Ireland 47, 50–1
  Southwark 79–82; *79*, *80*, *81*
Audit Commission 12, 14, 17, 30, 58

Balderton Hospital, Newark 41
Ballynahinch, Northern Ireland 51
Bamford, Margaret 44, 45–7, 50
Barker, Bill 40
Bassetlaw, Nottinghamshire 32–42
baths, home 4
Belfast 43–9
  City Hospital 43
Bevercotes Colliery 32
Beynon, Jan 27, 30
Blaenau, Gwent 21
Bottomley, Virginia 3
Bower, Joan 37–8
Boyd, Rene 44
Boyle, Lynn 63–4
Brewis, Alistair 58–9
British Medical Association 17
Browning, David 12
Burnett, Susan 27

Camberwell 83
care management 7–9, 10–11, 17
  Bassetlaw 33-5
  for disabled people 97–9
  monitoring 99–101
  Newcastle 61–4
  Southwark 77–80; *79*, *80*, *81*
care packages 61, 97–9
carers 29, 38, 50, 115–16
  Northern Ireland 48–9
  see also voluntary organisations
Carers National Association 48
Caring for People 77–8
case management 76–8, *78*
Case studies 8, 16, 98, 100
children
  disabled, cared for at home 48–9
  mentally handicapped 40, 53
Children Act 40
chiropody 69
Clark, Peter 26, 30
Claybury Hospital, Essex 107
Collis, Jean 40
community care services
  statistics 3
  timetable *14*
  see also contracts; health services; social services
Community Care Support Force 109
community health services *see* health services
community psychiatric nurses 35, 39
complaints 100
computer programs 24–5
consultation with users 109–10
contracts for social care 69–75, *73*
  monitoring 74, *74*
Costello, Julian 28
Counsel and Care 120
Crieff workshop 94
Crossroads 100

dementia 38
  Northern Ireland 51–2
  see also Alzheimer's disease
Department of Health 7, 17, 85
Department of Health and Social Services 43, 45–6, 51
Department of Social Security 92
Devon social services 69–75
  East Devon 101–3
Dingleton Hospital, Scotland 90
disabled people 109

121

INDEX

home care 16, 98, 100
  child 48–9
multiple sclerosis 8, 98, 100
Northern Ireland, statistics 44
statistics 3
user's view of care 96–104
Disabled Person's Act 1986   111
district nursing 4, 36, 69
doctors 12–13
  hospital 9
  see also general practitioners
Dodgson, Clare 56, 65
Dornan, Brian 47–8
Dowdeswell, Barry 58
Down and Lisburn management unit, Northern Ireland 47, 49–51, 52
Downshire Hospital 52
drug misusers 16, 84
Dunmurry, Northern Ireland 47, 50–1

East Devon 101–3
Eastgate Centre, Worksop 41
elderly people
  Bassetlaw 37–8
  home care 119–20
  Northern Ireland 49–52
  mentally infirm 51–2
  see also geriatrics; residential care
Exeter, East Devon 101, 103
Extra Care 51

Fairclough, Frances 35
Frazer of Carmyllie, Lord 88
Freeman, Ann 26–7, 28–9
Friern Hospital, north London 107, 108
fundholding 4, 8, 35–6, 64–5, 69–75, 84
funding 4–5, 9–10, 14–15, 86
  Newcastle 61–6, 62
  Northern Ireland 45–6, 47–8, 51
  residential homes 9, 22–3, 33, 46, 62, 84–5

Gartloch Asylum 91
Gartnavel Royal Hospital 90
Gellatly, Monica 36
general practitioners 8
  Bassetlaw 35–6
  fundholders 4, 8, 35–6, 64–5, 69–75
  Gwent 27–8
  Newcastle 61, 64
  Scotland 94
  training 64, 94
geriatrics 28–9, 34–5
  hospitals 26–7, 50–1

psychogeriatrics 25–6, 29, 38
statistics 3
Gibson, Joy 33, 39
Goodall, Trevor 39–40
Griffiths, Sir Roy 14, 77
Griffiths report 14–15
Gwent 21–31, *22*

handicap *see* disabled people; learning disability
Harvey, John 56–7, 65–6
health care 3–4, 10–11
Health of the Nation, The 24
health services 3
  Gwent 24
  relations with social services 69–72, 74, 75, 86–7
  Newcastle 64–5
  Northern Ireland 43–4
  screening 24, 28–9, 30
health visitors 74, 75
Hillhall Home, Lisburn 53
home care 4
  disabled people 8, 16, 98, 100
  child 48–9
  elderly people 49–50, 119–20
  Newcastle 57–8, 62
Hospital Services for the Mentally Ill 90–1
hospitals
  contracts 72
  discharge arrangements 6, 9–10, 16, 27, 34–5
  geriatric 26–7, 50–1
  Newcastle 58–9
  Northern Ireland 50–1
  Southwark 82
  doctors 9
  Newcastle 58
  NHS trusts 36–7, 44
  psychiatric 25–6, 39, 41, 51–2
  Scotland 89–90, 92–4
  user's view 106–12
hostels 92
House of Commons
  health committee 3
  social services committee 77
housing, for disabled people 97
Hunter, Stephen 25–6

Independent Living Fund (ILF) 8, 9, 98, 100
Inland Revenue 63
Italy, Law 180, 1978   92

INDEX

Ivybridge Health Centre *73*

Jenkins, Patricia 48
Jones, Maxwell 90
Jones, Peter 28

Larbert Asylum 93
learning disability (mental handicap) 12
  Bassetlaw 40–1
  children 40, 53
  Northern Ireland 52–4
  statistics 3
Lewis, Caroline 24–5
Living Options 96, 100, 101–3
local authorities
  funding 9, 14–15
  NHS, relations 6, 7, 10–11
  Northern Ireland 43, 44
  social care responsibilities 3–4, 6–7, 14–15, 80
    assessments 7
    consultation 109
    implementation 10
Lomax, Tess 71–2, 75
Love, Bill 48, 49

Manton Colliery 32
Marriot, Caroline 52–4
Marston, Jackie 59
May, Ann *28*, 29
McBrien, Mary 50–1
Mencap Homes Foundation 41
mental handicap *see* learning disability
Mental Health Act 1983   82, 85, 108
mental health and illness 12, 16
  Bassetlaw 33–4, 35, 39–41
  case management 76–8
  psychiatric nurses 35, 39
  Scotland 88–95
  Southwark 76–7
  statistics 3
  user's view 105–20
  see also hospitals, psychiatric
Mental Health in Focus 91
Mental Health (Scotland) Act 1984   92
Mental Health Task Force 109
Mental Illness Specific Grant 88
Meredith, Paul 22
MIND 25, 40, 109
Monmouth, Gwent 21, 23
Moody, Lynn 38
Moore, Bob 44, 45–6
Morris, Rhidian 69
Muckamore Abbey Hospital 52–4

Mullins, Julie 24
multiple sclerosis 8, 98, 100
Muthiah, M M 38

Napsbury Hospital, St Albans 90
Narayana, C L 41
National Health Service (NHS) 5–6, 10–11, 70
  trusts 36–7, 44
National Health Service and Community Care Act 1990   5–6, 45, 78, 82, 107
National Schizophrenia Fellowship 106, 109
needs 87
  see also assessment
Newcastle upon Tyne 55–66
  community care plan *65*
  expenditure *62*
  mental health consumer group 109–10
Newport, Gwent 21, 26–9
night sitting service 62
Northern Ireland 43–54
Nottinghamshire 32–42
nursing
  contracts 69–70, 75
  district 4, 36, 69
  psychiatric 35, 39
nursing homes *see* residential care

occupational therapy 36

patch teams 47, 49–51
Pathways to Quality Services 103
Pathy, John 27, 29–30
People First 45
Peysner, Penny 38
physical handicap *see* disabled people
Plymouth Community Trust 75
Plymouth Health Authority 71
Pratt, Peter 36, 41–2
Princess Royal Trust for Carers 49
psychiatric care *see* mental health and illness
psychogeriatrics 25–6, 29, 38
purchasing 66, 85–6

Rampton 39
Ranby prison 39
Reed report 39
Reeks, Jane 27
Relatives Association 113, 116–20
residential care and nursing homes *2*
  Bassetlaw 33, 34–5, 37, 38
  cost 83, 119

123

INDEX

funding 5, 9, 22–3, 33, 84–5
Newcastle 61–2
Northern Ireland 49
private 5, 9, 22–3, 92
relative's view 113–20
Southwark 83–5
Retford, Nottinghamshire 32, 41
Royal Edinburgh Hospital 90
Royal Victoria Infirmary, Newcastle 58–9
Roycroft, Brian 55–6, 58, 64, 66
Ruffell, Tony 35–6

Sands, Karen 41
Sangwin, Terry 59
Scotland, community psychiatric care 88–95
Scottish Health Authorities Priorities for the Eighties (SHAPE) 91, 93
Scottish Health Authorities Review of Priorities for the Eighties and Nineties (SHARPEN) 91, 93
Shearer, Raymond 45, 48
Sighthill health centre, Edinburgh 90
Silcock, Ben 105
Simpson, Rosemary 52
Smith, Gary 56, 58
social security benefits 5
social services
  inspectorate 78
  relations with health services 69–72, 74, 75, 86–7
  Newcastle 64–5
  Northern Ireland 43–4
social workers, teams 70–2
Southwark 76–87
  mental health services 76–7, 79–87
St Cadoc's hospital, Caerleon 25
St Woolos Hospital, Newport 26–7
Stephenson, Carolyn 61–3

Steven, Joyce 23
Survivors Speak Out 105

TEC-SYS program 24–5
training 69, 94
Tredegar, Gwent 23, 24–5, 30
trusts, NHS 36–7, 44
Turning Point 16, 39

United States of America 10
  Community Mental Health Centers Act 76
users
  disabled, provision for 96–104
  mental health services 105–12

voluntary organisations 109
  Age Concern 27, 37–8
  Bassetlaw 40
  distribution 84
  funding 63
  Gwent 27
  monitoring 100–1
  Northern Ireland 51
  see also carers

Walker, Jim 39
Walters, Frankie 56, 64–5
Warner, Nick 25–6, 29
Weightman, Kate 59–60
Welsh Office 21, 27
wheelchair services 102
Whitaker, Chris 71, 75
White, Denis 50, 51
Williams, Perry 24
Williams, Idris 36
Wilson, Anne 59
Worksop, Nottinghamshire 32, 35, 36–7, 39, 41